Handbook of

Vascular Surgery

Handbook of
Vascular Surgery

EDITED BY

Clifford M. Sales, M.D.
Attending Staff, Department of Surgery,
Overlook Hospital, Summit, New Jersey; and
Saint Barnabas Medical Center,
Livingston, New Jersey

Jamie Goldsmith, R.N.
Associate in Surgery and Patient Care
Coordinator, Vascular Surgical Services, Albert Einstein
College of Medicine, Montefiore Medical Center,
New York, New York

Frank J. Veith, M.D.
Professor and Chief, Vascular Surgical Services,
Albert Einstein College of Medicine, Montefiore Medical Center,
New York, New York

with 95 illustrations

Quality Medical Publishing, Inc.

ST. LOUIS, MISSOURI
1994

Printed in the United States of America.

PUBLISHER   Karen Berger
EDITOR   Beth Campbell
PROJECT MANAGER   Suzanne Seeley Wakefield
PRODUCTION   Susan Trail
BOOK DESIGN   Susan Trail
COVER DESIGN   Diane Beasley Design

Quality Medical Publishing, Inc.
11970 Borman Drive, Suite 222
St. Louis, Missouri 63146

LIBRARY OF CONGRESS CATALOGING-IN-PUBLICATION DATA

Handbook of vascular surgery / edited by Clifford M. Sales, Jamie
    Goldsmith, Frank J. Veith.
        p.   cm.
    Includes bibliographical references and index.
    ISBN 0-942219-49-X
    1. Blood-vessels—Surgery—Handbooks, manuals, etc.   2. Blood
-vessels—Diseases—Handbooks, manuals, etc.   I. Sales, Clifford M.
II. Goldsmith, Jamie.   III. Veith, Frank J.
    [DNLM: 1. Vascular Surgery—methods—handbooks.   2. Vascular
Diseases—surgery—handbooks.   WG 39 H2367 1994]
RD598.5.H364   1994
617.4'13—dc20
DNLM / DLC
for Library of Congress   94-9401
                                                               CIP

TH/RP/RP
5   4   3   2

Contributors

Norwin H. Becker, M.D.
Professor of Pathology, Albert Einstein College of Medicine, Montefiore Medical Center, New York, New York

George L. Berdejo, B.A., R.V.T.
Technical Director, Vascular Laboratory, Montefiore Medical Center, Bronx, New York

Hannah L. Brooks, M.D.
Chief Resident in Surgery, Albert Einstein College of Medicine, Montefiore Medical Center, New York, New York

Keith D. Calligaro, M.D.
Associate Clinical Professor of Surgery, Pennsylvania Hospital, University of Pennsylvania School of Medicine, Philadelphia, Pennsylvania

Alan M. Dietzek, M.D.
Assistant Professor of Surgery, Cornell University Medical College, Ithaca, New York

Elizabeth A. Farrell, PA-C
Clinical Coordinator, Division of Vascular Surgery, Albert Einstein College of Medicine, Montefiore Medical Center, New York, New York

Charles D. Franco, M.D.
Division of Vascular Surgery, St. Peter's Medical Center, and Robert Wood Johnson University Hospital, New Brunswick, New Jersey

Jamie Goldsmith, R.N.
Associate in Surgery and Patient Care Coordinator, Vascular Surgical Services, Albert Einstein College of Medicine, Montefiore Medical Center, New York, New York

Ross T. Lyon, M.D.
Assistant Professor of Surgery, Albert Einstein College of Medicine, Montefiore Medical Center, New York, New York

Michael L. Marin, M.D.
Assistant Professor of Surgery, Albert Einstein College of Medicine, Montefiore Medical Center, New York, New York

Ben U. Marsan, M.D.
Resident in General Surgery, Flushing Hospital Medical Center, Flushing, New York

Arthur T. Martella, M.D.
Chief Resident in Surgery, Albert Einstein College of Medicine, Montefiore Medical Center, New York, New York

Thomas F. Panetta, M.D.
Professor of Surgery and Radiology, Chief of Vascular Surgery, State University of New York, Health Science Center at Brooklyn, Brooklyn, New York

Amit V. Patel, M.D.
Fellow in Vascular Surgery, University of Pennsylvania, Philadelphia, Pennsylvania

Clifford M. Sales, M.D.
Attending Staff, Department of Surgery, Overlook Hospital, Summit, New Jersey; and Saint Barnabas Medical Center, Livingston, New Jersey

Luis A. Sanchez, M.D.
Fellow in Vascular Surgery, Albert Einstein College of Medicine, Montefiore Medical Center, New York, New York

Larry A. Scher, M.D.
Director of Vascular Surgery, North Shore University Hospital;
Associate Professor of Surgery, Cornell University Medical College,
Ithaca, New York

Michael L. Schwartz, M.D.
Fellow in Vascular Surgery, Albert Einstein College of Medicine,
Montefiore Medical Center, New York, New York

Michael B. Silva, Jr., M.D.
Fellow in Vascular Surgery, University of Medicine and Dentistry
of New Jersey, Newark, New Jersey

William D. Suggs, M.D.
Assistant Professor of Surgery, Albert Einstein College of Medicine,
Montefiore Medical Center, New York, New York

Frank J. Veith, M.D.
Professor and Chief, Vascular Surgical Services, Albert Einstein
College of Medicine, Montefiore Medical Center, New York, New
York

Kurt R. Wengerter, M.D.
Assistant Professor of Surgery, Albert Einstein College of Medicine,
Montefiore Medical Center, New York, New York

Preface

The maturation of vascular surgery into a specialty has allowed for the rapid expansion of the fund of knowledge of diseases of the cardiovascular system. This information explosion has provided a better understanding of the mechanisms of atherosclerosis and other vascular disease processes. Vascular surgeons have played a significant role in elucidating the basic scientific mechanisms underlying these disease processes—a testament to the commitment of practitioners of this specialty.

The field of vascular surgery, although involved in the basic mechanisms of atherogenesis and other vascular diseases, is primarily a clinical specialty. Restoration of unobstructed laminar blood flow remains central to most vascular surgical procedures. Successful outcomes in these procedures demand not only accurate diagnosis and selection of the correct surgical procedure but also flawless execution of the chosen operation in a consistent manner. Surgical technique cannot be learned from a book; hence we have intentionally omitted in-depth technical descriptions from this book. The basic techniques necessary for performing these operations are currently taught in vascular surgery training programs.

Handbook of Vascular Surgery highlights some important aspects of the diagnosis and management of vascular disease. It has not been designed as a textbook of vascular surgery, nor is it meant to be all inclusive. Rather, the reader will gain a basis for understanding a particular problem and some of the alternatives for its management. This book will provide a foundation of information that can, if necessary, stimulate further exploration of the topic in the referenced literature and more detailed vascular texts.

The rapid evolution of this field makes it impossible to cover all of the important topics encountered in vascular surgery. Many of the "cutting edge" advances and less common disease processes have been omitted to allow space for the more common vascular problems. Understandably, any book reflects the bias of its creators. Although a generally "standard" approach has been presented throughout, certain biases are still present. Most contributors to *Handbook* have been trained in the art and science of vascular surgery by the senior editor. Thus the views presented herein represent the teaching of our vascular surgical group and reflect the testing of these lessons by a long experience in the field.

Handbook is intended to serve a multitude of health care providers well with its straightforward, problem-based approach. Maturing surgeons in training will find the basics with which to approach a specific vascular surgical problem, alerting them to the salient diagnostic points and treatment plans. Established physicians will now have a concise reference so that many of the less obvious points regarding their patient's diagnosis and treatment plans can be recalled. Nursing personnel, interns, and allied health professionals can derive a basic understanding of disease processes and management strategies.

The contributions of all of the authors remain the heart of this book. Their intellect and diligence are reflected in the pages of *Handbook of Vascular Surgery*. A sincere thanks is extended to Michael Torres, whose photographic contributions have been invaluable. Another important person in producing this book is Maxine D'Amelio. Her dedication, insight, and resourcefulness in editing and preparing manuscripts have earned our deepest appreciation.

Clifford M. Sales
Jamie Goldsmith
Frank J. Veith

Contents

Handbook of

Vascular Surgery

1

Basic Science of Vascular Disease

Michael L. Marin • Frank J. Veith • Norwin H. Becker

Largely as a result of advancements over the past 30 years, vascular surgery has evolved into a unique specialty. Vascular imaging modalities and surgical techniques have been improved, and there are new developments in endoluminal therapies and vascular graft technology. A greater understanding of the basic mechanisms of vascular pathology has further advanced vascular medicine. With future investigations of the primary mechanisms of atherosclerosis, cellular proliferation, and coagulation, more effective treatments for vascular disease will evolve.

Vascular Wall Microanatomy

ARTERIES. The arterial wall consists of three concentric layers: (1) the inner layer *(intima)* is a tube of endothelial cells in which the long axis of each cell is oriented longitudinally; (2) the middle layer *(media)* is composed predominantly of circumferentially arranged smooth muscle cells—the intima and media are separated from each other by the *internal elastic lamina;* and (3) the outer layer *(adventitia)* consists of fibroblasts and connective tissue that is loosely incorporat-

1

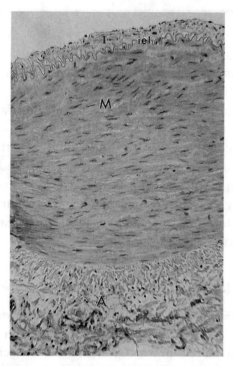

Fig. 1-1. Light micrograph of a normal-appearing anterior tibial artery from a 23-year-old man following traumatic amputation. The three distinct layers of the artery wall can be discerned. (*I* = intima; *M* = media; *A* = adventitia; *iel* = internal elastic lamina.)

ed into the connective tissue surrounding the vessel (Fig. 1-1). The media and adventitial layers are separated by a dense fibrous element known as the *external elastic lamina*.

VEINS. Veins transport blood from capillary beds and increase in caliber and wall thickness as they progress toward the heart. While three distinct layers exist in the walls of veins (intima, media, adventitia), the boundaries between these layers are less distinct than in the arterial system. With the exception of muscular veins (such as the greater saphenous vein), the vein wall media is virtually indistinguishable from the extensive connective tissue component of the vein walls (Fig. 1-2).

Most medium-sized veins (greater than 2.5 mm in diameter) in the extremities contain valves that direct the flow of blood toward the heart. Valves appear as semilunar pockets on the internal surface of the vein wall. The valve leaflets are arranged in pairs so as to appose one another. Each valve is a thin connective tissue membrane containing elastic fibers within its intima and its surfaces are covered by endothelium (Fig. 1-3).

LYMPHATICS. The lymphatic vessels provide a secondary drainage conduit for protein, water, and electrolytes contained in the extravascular environment.

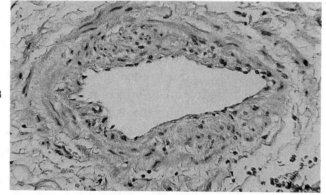

Fig. 1-2. A, Light micrograph of a greater saphenous vein. Extensive medial smooth muscle composed of an inner longitudinal (M^1) and an outer circular (M^2) component can be seen in this muscular vein. **B,** Many veins in the human vasculature contain minimal medial smooth muscles, as seen here in this light micrograph of a branch of the posterior tibial vein.

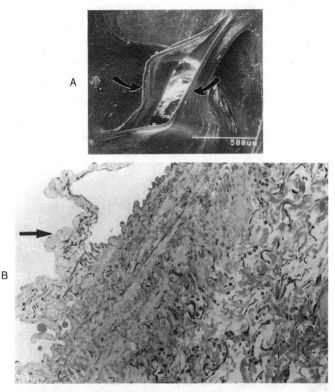

Fig. 1-3. A, Scanning electron micrograph of a saphenous vein branch valve. Vein valves are typically semilunar structures that anchor to the medial layer of the vein (*arrows* show valve leaflets). **B,** Light micrograph of a saphenous vein valve *(arrow).* Continuity with the inner layer of medial smooth muscle is apparent.

The peripheral lymphatics are frequently encountered by vascular surgeons in the management of primary and secondary lymphedema (see Chapter 14). The microscopic anatomy of peripheral lymphatic vessels greater than 0.2 mm in diameter demonstrates three layers corresponding to intima, media and adventitia (Fig. 1-4). The borders between these layers are poorly defined. Valves are conspicuous features of lymphatic vessels and are usually paired and extremely thin.

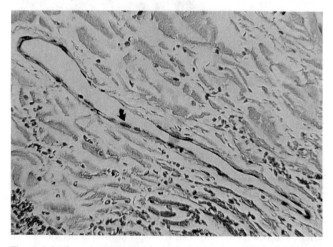

Fig. 1-4. Light micrograph of a lymphatic vessel that runs along the course of the posterior tibial artery. The walls are thin, with a single endothelial layer visible *(arrow)*.

Mechanisms of Vascular Disease

Destruction of the normal architecture of the vascular wall often results in clinically apparent disease. The stimulus for such disturbances in normal vessel structure and function may be caused by inflammation, atherosclerosis or the sequelae of vascular thrombosis.

ATHEROSCLEROSIS

Etiologic factors. Atherosclerosis is a pathologic process characterized by the accumulation of cells, lipids, and matrix fibers (plaque) in the intima of large arteries. The progression of this degenerative process produces narrowing of the vessel lumen. This causes obstruction of the flow of blood, ulceration, embolization and, eventually, thrombosis. Although atherosclerosis is a systemic disorder, plaque deposition occurs with greater frequency at selected sites within the arterial tree.

A number of etiologic factors have been identified for atherosclerosis; these include hyperlipidemia, hypertension, and certain viral infections. All of these produce endothelial cell injury, smooth muscle cell proliferation, and plaque formation. Altered local hemodynamic conditions, such as turbulent flow at arterial bifurcations, produce low and/or oscillatory wall shear stress, which can result in vessel wall injury and the development of atherosclerotic plaque.

Pathologic anatomy. Fibrous plaque is the predominant lesion of atherosclerosis (Fig. 1-5). Plaques are usually eccentric and are commonly composed of endothelium overlying poorly differentiated smooth muscle cells, connective tissues, and mononuclear cells.

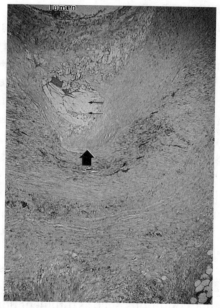

Fig. 1-5. Light micrograph of an atherosclerotic plaque contained within a popliteal artery from an amputated limb. A relatively acellular cap *(arrow)* is seen, with cholesterol and calcification in the deep portion of the plaque *(double arrow).*

Frequently there is a necrotic center of debris composed of dead cells, fibrous elements, and droplet forms of lipid. Lipid is also widely seen within the cytoplasm of the surrounding smooth muscle cells. Calcium salts are present in mature plaques and appear in crystalline form or as large plates.

ARTERIAL ANEURYSMS. Aneurysmal vascular disease refers to those events in the course of vascular wall pathology which result in the focal or diffuse dilatation of an artery. Etiologic factors that contribute to aneurysm formation may be categorized by their classic clinical description, as shown below.

Etiologic Classification of Arterial Aneurysms

Congenital	Medial agenesis
	Marfan's syndrome
	Ehlers-Danlos syndrome
	Genetic defects of elastin and collagen
Inflammatory	Syphilitic
	Bacterial
	Noninfectious inflammatory disease
Traumatic	Traumatic aneurysm
	Anastomotic (postsurgical)
	Poststenotic aneurysm
Degenerative	Arteriosclerotic
	Fibrodysplasia

Regardless of the precise cause, aneurysms form under two general conditions: (1) increased mechanical stress on the arterial wall and (2) decreased intrinsic strength and structural integrity of the arterial wall.

INTIMAL HYPERPLASIA. Arterial reconstruction has become the treatment of choice for the management of occlusive disease of small arteries of the heart, viscera, brain, and the extremities. Such bypasses usually employ autogenous veins as the ideal conduit; however, as many as 25% of these vein grafts will develop stenoses and ultimately thrombose.

The precise cause of failure of a bypass graft is often difficult to determine. One possible cause is that the narrowing of the lumen of a graft or endarterectomized artery may proceed by recurrent or progressive atherosclerosis, superimposed on normal wound healing. This process, called *intimal hyperplasia,* consists largely of the proliferation of smooth muscle cells and deposition of connective tissue within the intima (Fig. 1-6). The precise growth factors and inhibitors that regulate the balance between normal vessel healing and progression to pathologic stenosis remain unknown. Identification of these factors, along with an understanding of how they regulate smooth muscle cell growth, will likely lead to new forms of preventive therapy.

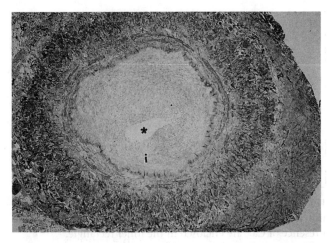

Fig. 1-6. Light micrograph of a saphenous vein graft stenosis. The lumen *(*)* is markedly reduced by the formation of extensive myointimal proliferation *(i)*.

HEMOSTASIS AND THROMBOSIS. Understanding the general mechanisms of coagulation is of great importance to the vascular surgeon, who frequently operates to correct the sequelae of thrombosis or who observes a vascular reconstruction made unsuccessful by a thrombotic complication. Hemostasis and thrombosis are processes that share the same orderly pathways but differ in that thrombosis results in coagulation that is excessive and/or occurs in an inappropriate location (Fig. 1-7).

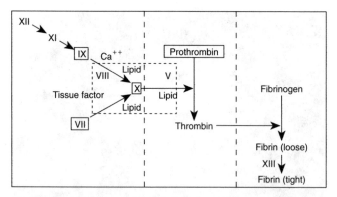

Fig. 1-7. The clotting mechanism. Factors in boxes require vitamin K to complete synthesis. Those reactions which require the presence of Ca^{++} are enclosed in the inner rectangle.

ANTICOAGULANTS. *Heparin* is a sulfated polysaccharide obtained from pork, beef lung, or beef intestine. Heparin catalyzes the inactivation of thrombin and factors XIIa, XIa, Xa, and IXa by antithrombin III. Heparin must be administered intravenously or subcutaneously, because it is not effectively absorbed from the intestinal tract. The half-life of heparin is 90 minutes. An important side effect of heparin, in addition to bleeding, is its ability to cause platelet clumping and thrombocytopenia. The effects of heparin can be immediately reversed by administering protamine sulfate at a dose of 1.0 to 1.5 mg per 100 µg of heparin.

Warfarin interferes with the vitamin K–dependent step in the synthesis of factors II, VII, IX, and X. When administered orally, warfarin's "therapeutic range" is usually approached within 36 hours. However, an increased responsiveness to warfarin occurs in patients with liver disease, congestive heart failure and hypothyroidism. The opposite effect, a muted response, is achieved by estrogen therapy, because the synthesis of vitamin K–dependent factors is increased.

ANTIPLATELET THERAPY. An enhanced understanding of platelet function has led to the development of new drugs that have the capacity to alter platelet activity. The drugs that have undergone the most extensive clinical trials include aspirin, dipyridamole, sulfinpyrazone and dextran.

Aspirin interferes with platelet function by irreversibly acetylating cyclo-oxygenase. A single 150 mg dose will result in defective platelet function for several days.

Dipyridamole inhibits the enzyme cyclic AMP phosphodiesterase and enhances the plasma level of the platelet inhibitor adenosine by blocking adenosine's uptake in red blood cells. It may also act by inhibiting thromboxane synthesis. Although commonly used in combination, synergy between dipyridamole and aspirin in inhibiting thrombosis has not been proven in clinical trials.

Sulfinpyrazone is a nonsteroidal anti-inflammatory drug (NSAID) that acts by reversibly inhibiting cyclo-oxygenase. Successful clinical trials have been reported.

Dextran is a branched polysaccharide, produced in two molecular weight forms (dextran 40 and dextran 70), with apparent equal antithrombotic action. The precise mode of action of dextran is not known; however, it has been shown to increase the speed of clot lysis (altered fibrin polymerization) as well as depress platelet aggregation and adhesiveness.

BIBLIOGRAPHY

Anidjar S, Kieffer E. Pathogenesis of acquired aneurysms. Ann Vasc Surg 6:298-305, 1992.

Anticoagulation. Chest 95 (suppl): 2, 1989.

Bloom W, Fawcett DW. A Textbook of Histology. Philadelphia: WB Saunders, 1975.

Halleh JW, Jr. Abdominal aortic aneurysms: Natural history and treatment. Heart Dis Stroke 1:303-308, 1992.

Svensson L, Crawford S. Aortic dissection and aortic aneurysm surgery: Clinical observations, experimental investigations and statistical analysis, parts I and II. Current Probl Surg 29:11-12, 1992.

Svensson L, Crawford S. Aortic dissection and aortic aneurysm surgery: Clinical observations, experimental investigations and statistical analysis, part III. Current Probl Surg 30:1, 1993.

Varty K, Allen KE, Bell PRF, et al. Infrainguinal vein graft stenosis. Br J Surg 80:825-833, 1993.

White RA, ed. Atherosclerosis and Arteriosclerosis: Human Pathology and Experimental Animal Methods and Models. Boca Raton, Fla: CRC Press, 1989.

2
History and Physical Examination

Michael L. Schwartz

The value of a history and physical examination should not be underestimated in establishing a correct diagnosis. This part of the patient evaluation also builds the foundation on which further diagnostic tests and therapeutic interventions may be planned.

Peripheral Vascular Disease

HISTORY. Pain is the most common chief complaint regardless of whether the occlusive disease is acute or chronic. Pain may present as either intermittent claudication or pain at rest.

Intermittent claudication, derived from the Latin *claudico,* meaning "to limp," is a pain that is brought on by exercise and relieved with rest. It is typically described as a cramping sensation or a feeling of tiredness. It is reproducible by the same level of exercise and is relieved by rest within 2 to 5 minutes. Occasionally a patient may describe a sensation of heaviness, weakness, or fatigue in the limb without pain.

The pathophysiology of claudication is that of muscle ischemia caused by diminished oxygen delivery. An occlusion or stenosis of the arteries supplying a particular muscle group will limit flow; therefore the increased metabolic demands during exercise cannot be met.

Most patients with calf claudication have an occlusion of the superficial femoral artery. Bilateral thigh or buttock claudication associated with erectile dysfunction is known as the *Leriche syndrome.* The impotence is the result of inadequate blood flow through the hypogastric artery.

When assessing a patient who has claudication, it is important to question the duration, severity, and progression of the symptoms. Severity is most reliably assessed by the number of city blocks the patient can ambulate before claudication begins. It is also important to assess the degree of disability the condition imposes on the patient.

Ischemic rest pain is easily differentiated from claudication. Rest pain is a constant pain described as a severe aching or burning in the foot. The pain usually localizes to the metatarsal heads but may be worse in the location of a gangrenous toe or ischemic ulcer. This pain often intensifies at night and may be relieved by dependency (that is, hanging the foot over the side of the bed).

Rest pain is of far greater consequence than is claudication. Whereas the latter may remain a benign condition, rest pain heralds the onset of gangrene and demands immediate attention.

Symptoms of spinal stenosis, sciatica, osteoarthritis, or causalgia may be indistinguishable from those of vasculogenic claudication, hence the name "pseudo-claudication." However, these patients have intact peripheral pulses without other evidence of vascular disease. Diabetic neuropathy is another diagnosis frequently confused with ischemic rest pain. Diabetic neuropathy is not relieved by changes in position, and the patient lacks the associated physical findings of peripheral vascular disease (PVD).

Ambulatory status. The ability to ambulate before the onset of PVD must be ascertained to develop an effective therapeutic approach. Nonambulatory patients with organic brain syndrome or neuromuscular disorders should be considered for primary amputation in the face of a threatened limb. However, patients who do not ambulate but use their limb for transferring or other activities of daily living should be considered for revascularization. The loss of a limb in these patients may cause them to become bedridden.

Risk factors. Smoking is probably the most important contributing factor to PVD. Smoking accelerates the atherosclerotic process and causes vasospasm. It also has been shown to decrease the patency of vascular reconstructions. The patient's smoking history should be quantitated in pack-years (number of packs per day multiplied by the number of years).

Diabetes mellitus is present in more than 70% of the patients with vascular disease at our institution.

Hypertension and hyperlipidemia are also contributing risk factors of PVD. Although renal insufficiency is a result of atherosclerosis and not a risk factor for PVD, it has been shown that patients with end-stage renal disease are at a higher risk for limb loss even in the presence of a patent vascular reconstruction. Other manifestations of the atherosclerotic disease process, such as coronary artery and cerebrovascular disease, must be specifically sought out. A list of the patient's medications must be obtained, with special attention to the use of insulin, oral hypoglycemic agents, antihypertensives, anticoagulants, and corticosteroids. Allergies to medications as well as to shellfish and iodine should be noted. The patient's surgical history must be ascertained, with emphasis on previous lower extremity revascularizations or coronary artery bypass procedures in which a saphenous vein graft was used. Previous operations for varicose veins or a past history of phlebitis should be noted, because this may render the veins unsuitable for use in bypass grafting.

PHYSICAL EXAMINATION. The physical examination should be carried out in an organized fashion so that important aspects are not overlooked. *Gross inspection* for swelling, color changes, trophic changes, ulceration, or gangrene must be performed.

Swelling (edema) may be caused by congestive heart failure, venous valvular incompetence, inflammation, or lymphedema.

Color changes should be carefully described. A blue, dusky extremity may signify a threatened limb. *Dependent rubor* is pallor of the skin of the foot when the leg is elevated that returns to a bright red color when the leg is dependent.

Trophic changes are noted in the skin, hair, and nails of the foot. The skin of a patient with PVD may appear thin, pale, and shiny. There is often no hair on the feet or toes. The toenails are rough and thickened as a result of retarded growth.

Lower extremity ulceration may be neuropathic, arterial, or venous in origin (Table 2-1). The typical venous stasis ulcer is found over the medial malleolus in association with brawny pigmentation of the skin (such as stasis dermatitis). It may be painful and when debrided will bleed. Neuropathic or malperforans ulcers are painless lesions often found on the heel or under the metatarsal heads. They bleed briskly when debrided. Arterial ulcers are very painful and are associated with manifestations of PVD. Debridement results in minimal bleeding. These lesions often have a necrotic base and can be found distally on the dorsum of the foot or toes. It should be noted that some ulcerations have a mixed arteriovenous or arterial and neuropathic component. This determination can be made by the pulse examination.

Table 2-1. Differential Diagnosis of Leg Ulceration

Parameter	Arterial	Venous	Neuropathic
Location	Foot	Ankle	Metatarsal heads, weight-bearing surfaces
Pain	Severe	Mild to moderate	None
Ulcer bed	Fibrinous exudate, necrosis	Fibrinous exudate, granulation tissue	Granulation tissue, callus
Associated findings	Trophic changes	Stasis dermatitis	Abnormal sensation
Pulse examination	Diminished	Present	Usually present

Gangrene refers to tissue necrosis. The blackened tissue is insensate and often hard and shriveled. A line of demarcation may exist between viable and nonviable tissue.

Palpation of the extremity involves assessment of the gross temperature as well as the presence of masses. To quantitate temperature changes, the examiner should expose the limb to the ambient environment for at least 5 minutes, and the limbs must be compared with one another.

Pulse examination is the most important part of the physical examination. The performance of a careful pulse examination can provide an accurate assessment of the lower extremity circulation. Besides palpation of the carotid, brachial, and radial pulses, the common femoral, popliteal, and pedal pulses should be assessed. The pulses should be graded in a standard fashion (Table 2-2).

Table 2-2. Standard Pulse Examination

Grade	Characteristic
0	Absent
1+	Diminished*
2+	Normal
3+	Accentuated, aneurysmal

*Confirmed by counting pulse out loud while another examiner simultaneously counts an easily palpable pulse (such as the radial pulse).

Accurate pulse examination should be done in a consistent manner. The patient should be supine and motionless. Both arms should be at the patient's side and the patient should be undressed or wearing loose-fitting clothes.

The common femoral artery is found midway between the pubic tubercle and the anterior superior iliac spine. For pulses that are difficult to feel, the application of gradually increasing pressure may be helpful. The popliteal pulse is best felt with the patient's knee in full extension. The examiner places both hands in the middle of the popliteal fossa with the fingers lined up next to each other. The palms of the hand may be cupped or in contact with the patient's knee. If the pulse is difficult to feel, the knee may be slightly flexed. The pedal pulses are often difficult to feel, and the search for these pulses should be carried out in a relaxed, unhurried fashion. The dorsalis pedis pulse is found between the first and second metatarsals. Dorsiflexion of the ankle may make the pulse more easily palpable. The posterior tibial artery is located just posterior to the medial malleolus.

Based on the vascular history and physical examination, the patient's arterial disease may be classified into one of five stages of ischemia (Table 2-3).

Table 2-3. Stages of Ischemia

Stage	Presentation
0	No signs or symptoms
1	Intermittent claudication (>1 block)
2	Severe claudication (<½ block)
3	Rest pain
4	Ischemic ulcer or gangrene

Aortic Aneurysmal Disease

HISTORY. Most abdominal aortic aneurysms (AAAs) are asymptomatic and are detected during physical examination or evaluation of other disease processes. Unfortunately, some patients learn of the presence of an aneurysm only after they are admitted to the hospital with a ruptured aneurysm. In any patient presenting with the acute onset of abdominal, back, flank, or groin pain a diagnosis of ruptured AAA must be considered.

Several genetic studies suggest that AAAs are a familial disease, and a careful history may reveal the presence of AAA in another family member. Identification of a patient with AAA disease and a female relative with an aneurysm strongly correlates with the risk of rupture—the so-called ***black widow syndrome.***

PHYSICAL EXAMINATION. The success of palpating an abdominal aortic aneurysm depends on the patient's body habitus. This can be difficult in an obese patient. The experienced examiner can reliably determine the size of the aorta in a lean patient; however, it is often overestimated. An AAA is felt as a pulsatile mass in the abdomen above the umbilicus and often to the left of the patient's midline. The proper technique is bimanual examination with fairly light palpation. Both hands are usually pushed laterally by the pulsation of the aneurysm if present. If a pulsatile mass is felt below the umbilicus, associated iliac artery aneurysms should be considered.

A patient with an AAA has a 5% to 10% chance of having another aneurysm in the lower extremity. Sixty percent of patients with a popliteal aneurysm have an associated AAA.

Some patients with an AAA may present with abdominal pain or tenderness. This is found with ruptured, inflammatory, or infected aneurysms or in aneurysms that have recently undergone rapid expansion. Other diagnoses to be considered with pulsatile abdominal masses include pancreatic neoplasms or pseudocyst, horseshoe kidney, or retroperitoneal tumors.

Patients with an AAA may present with the classic *blue toe syndrome.* This is characterized by atheroemboli from the aorta occluding the digital vessels of the foot. These patients have ischemic toes with palpable pulses. Radiographic assessment of the patient's aortoiliac system is mandatory.

Cerebrovascular Disease

HISTORY. Cerebrovascular disease may be asymptomatic. The manifestations may range from brief episodes of neurologic dysfunction (transient ischemic attack) to permanent neurologic defects from stroke. A transient ischemic attack (TIA) consists of a neurologic deficit, with complete resolution in less than 24 hours. Most TIAs last for only a few minutes and are the result of microemboli from carotid atherosclerotic disease. It is associated with a stroke risk of almost 40% within 5 years. A majority of these strokes will occur during the first year after the TIA.

A specific type of TIA, amaurosis fugax, results from microembolization of the first branch of the internal carotid artery, the ophthalmic artery. The patient describes a transient loss of vision in one eye, likened to a "shade or curtain closing." The combination of amaurosis fugax and contralateral TIAs essentially confirms the diagnosis of cerebral embolic disease.

Vertebrobasilar insufficiency produces a less well defined set of symptoms. Patients may complain of vertigo, diplopia, dysphagia, or disequilibrium. These symptoms are frequently bilateral. *Subclavian steal syndrome* refers to the reversal of flow in the ipsilateral vertebral artery to supply the distal subclavian artery in the presence of a proximal subclavian obstruction. Patients with this condition experience vertebrobasilar symptoms in response to exercise of the ipsilateral arm.

PHYSICAL EXAMINATION. The common carotid artery is the only extracranial cerebral artery able to be palpated directly. The presence of a pulse in the superficial temporal artery confirms patency of the external carotid artery.

The subclavian artery pulse is palpable in the neck just superior to the middle of the clavicle. A pulse in the axillary artery confirms patency of the subclavian artery.

Auscultation of the subclavian and carotid arteries is an integral part of the examination. The stethoscope is placed midway between the mastoid process and the sternal notch. The patient is asked to hold a deep breath while the examiner listens for bruits. The presence of a bruit may represent a stenosis in the vessel proximal to where the bruit is heard. However, the absence of a bruit may signify either no stenosis or a very high-grade stenosis or occlusion. The heart is also carefully auscultated, because a bruit may be, in fact, a transmitted cardiac murmur. A funduscopic examination may reveal the presence of emboli, visible as small, bright flecks (Hollenhorst plaques). This atheromatous debris is often lodged at the bifurcation of retinal arterioles.

In the examination of a patient with cerebrovascular disease, a thorough neurologic examination must be performed. This includes a thorough assessment of the cranial nerves as well as a baseline sensorimotor evaluation of the extremities.

BIBLIOGRAPHY

Calligaro KD, Veith FJ. Proper technique of lower extremity pulse examination. Contemp Surg 40:49-51, 1992.

Connor J, Wilson SE, Williams RA. The clinical examination of the vascular system. In Wilson SE, Veith FJ, Hobson RW II, Williams RA, eds. Vascular Surgery, Principles and Practices. New York: McGraw-Hill, 1987, pp 70-79.

Marston A. The clinical evaluation of the patient with atheroma. In Bell PRF, Jamieson CW, Ruckley CV, eds. Surgical Management of Vascular Disease. London: WB Saunders Ltd, 1992, pp 119-130.

Rutherford RB. Initial clinical evaluation—the vascular consultation. In Rutherford RB, ed. Vascular Surgery. Philadelphia: WB Saunders, 1977, pp 3-13.

Veith FJ, Ascer E, Gupta S, Sprayregen S. Femoral-popliteal-tibial occlusive disease. In Moore WS, ed. Vascular Surgery: A Comprehensive Review, 2nd ed. New York: Grune & Stratton, 1986, pp 513-525.

Veith FJ, Gupta SK, Wengerter KR, Goldsmith J, Rivers SP, Bakal C, Dietzek AM, Cynamon J, Sprayregen S, Gliedman ML. Changing arteriosclerotic disease patterns and management strategies in lower-limb-threatening ischemia. Ann Surg 212:402-412, 1990.

3

Noninvasive Studies

Kurt R. Wengerter • George L. Berdejo

The clinician's need for anatomic and physiologic information beyond that acquired by physical examination has given the noninvasive vascular laboratory a central role in the management of vascular disease. The equipment initially available was quite limited, providing only pressure measurements and plethysmography. The introduction and development of advanced ultrasound equipment and other computerized imaging devices have greatly expanded the scope of noninvasive vascular testing. Today these devices can provide high-resolution imaging and accurate flow information. As a result, we are observing an erosion of the role of invasive contrast arteriography as the *definitive* vascular imaging modality.

Overview of Noninvasive Testing

Noninvasive testing can be divided into three separate modalities: pressure measurement, flow measurement, and imaging. Each contributes valuable information for the evaluation of vascular disease.

PRESSURE MEASUREMENT. Pressure measurement was one of the first means for evaluating the circulatory system. The sphygmomanometer, developed in the nineteenth century, functions by determining the pressure required to occlude a vessel. Segmental extremity pressure measurements are determined by inflating a pneumatic cuff, placed on the extremity, to a suprasystolic pressure. A Doppler probe is used to auscultate an artery distal to the cuff for return of flow as the pressure in the cuff is slowly released. The pressure at which flow returns is the systolic arterial pressure. The selection of a properly sized cuff is imperative to minimize the effect that extravascular tissue volume (fat and muscle) can have on the pressure measurement. The width of the cuff should be approximately 1.2 times the diameter of the extremity, and the bladder of the cuff (the component that holds the air inflated under pressure) should encircle the limb completely. When the cuff is *less* than 1.2 times the diameter of the limb, a greater amount of pressure is required to compress the underlying tissue and occlude the vessel, thereby producing a falsely *high* pressure reading. Conversely, when the cuff is too *large,* a falsely *low* pressure reading will be recorded. Arterial calcification can also produce a falsely *high* reading, since heavily calcified vessels resist compression and do not easily collapse under pressure. There are instances in which the vessel cannot be occluded at the maximum pressure tolerated by the patient.

FLOW MEASUREMENT

Plethysmography. Plethysmography measures volume changes corresponding to blood flow into and out of the extremity. Arterial plethysmography is used to measure the pulse volume, or the volume changes, of a portion of a limb during the cardiac cycle. Venous plethysmography is typically used to assess the rate of venous outflow at the calf level.

A number of plethysmographic methods are available, including water displacement, strain gauge, impedance, and air plethysmography. Water displacement plethysmography is cumbersome and is not used clinically. Although strain-gauge and impedance plethysmography are reliable and sensitive methods, they have been replaced by the more convenient air plethysmograph. In *air plethysmography,* first popularized in the pulse volume recorder (PVR) device, a pneumatic cuff is used to encircle the extremity. The cuff is inflated to 65 mm Hg, and a pressure transducer records pressure changes occurring during the cardiac cycle. At this low inflation pressure, changes in pressure are proportional to the volume changes within the tissue under the cuff. The output from these devices is usually semiquantitative, with the displayed waveform proportional to the volume changes. Air plethysmography is most helpful in assessing limb perfusion in patients with severe arterial calcification (such as patients with diabetes). The rigidity of arteries present in such conditions interferes with pressure measurement and leads to falsely high values. Plethysmography does not rely on the compression and occlusion of an artery and therefore is not affected by such calcification.

Ocular plethysmography (OPG) is used to measure the volume changes within the eye caused by the arterial pulsations. Two techniques have been developed, both of which were designed to provide information about clinically significant carotid artery disease. The Kartchner-McRae OPG method evaluates the *delay* in volume filling of the eye resulting from a proximal carotid artery stenosis—a *true* plethysmographic technique. The OPG-Gee method uses a vacuum applied to the sclera to determine the intraocular pressure. This is primarily a pressure measurement technique and *not* a true plethysmograph. The intraocular pressure measured by the OPG-Gee technique corresponds with the internal carotid artery pressure and therefore can be used to detect a carotid artery stenosis significant enough (>60% diameter reduction) to cause a drop in pressure. Both of these techniques are indirect tests of carotid artery stenoses and were extremely valuable before direct noninvasive means of carotid artery evaluation became available. Both have now largely been replaced by duplex ultrasonography for the routine assessment of extracranial cerebrovascular disease.

Photoplethysmography (PPG) is another *indirect* method for evaluating cutaneous blood flow. A photoelectric sensor measures light from a light-emitting diode reflected by red blood cells in the dermal microcirculation. Arterial pulsations and venous congestion will increase the amount of blood in the dermal circulation, and will, in turn, be measured by the photoelectric sensor.

Doppler. The Doppler flow detector is one of the most useful instruments available for assessing blood flow. Its function is based on the "Doppler effect," or the change in frequency of waves (sound or other) returning from a moving object (reflector) (Fig. 3-1). A reflector moving *away* from the Doppler probe sends sound waves back at a frequency *lower* than its native frequency, while a reflector moving *toward* the probe will *increase* the frequency of the returning sound waves. Red blood cells are the predominant reflectors in the cardiovascular system. The faster they are moving, the greater the frequency shift they produce. The change in frequency is determined by comparing the frequency of the generated ultrasound waves with the frequency of the returning ultrasound waves.

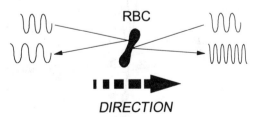

Fig. 3-1. Doppler effect. The frequency change of the reflected sound waves depends on the velocity of the reflector. In blood the predominant reflector is the red blood cell (RBC).

Two types of Doppler flow detectors are available. The ***continuous-wave Doppler probe*** continuously emits and receives ultrasound waves (Fig. 3-2). This requires both a sending and a receiving crystal in the probe. These crystals ***insonate,*** or send and receive Doppler signals from all structures within the range of the probe. Output is usually audio, and the experienced operator can distinguish between the higher pitched arterial signal and the lower pitched venous signal. Because the returning signals may include a combination of arterial and venous signals, the operator must

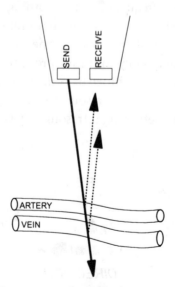

Fig. 3-2. Continuous-wave Doppler imaging. Sending and receiving crystals are continuously functioning. Doppler signals return from all structures insonated.

be able to recognize this and, if possible, separate the signals by redirecting the probe. Continuous-wave Doppler systems are generally more compact and portable than pulsed-wave units and are usually the type used in hand-held units.

The ***pulsed-wave Doppler flow detector*** emits ultrasound waves in pulses. The piezoelectric crystal is activated only for a brief period of time (Fig. 3-3) to send an ultrasound pulse and then is reactivated briefly to receive a returning signal. Most pulsed-wave Dopplers are combined with B-mode imaging (duplex scan-

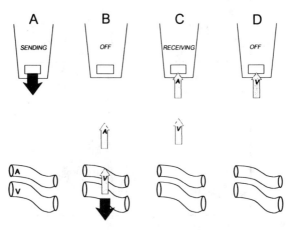

Fig. 3-3. Pulsed-wave Doppler imaging. **A**, Pulsed wave signal is sent. **B**, Crystal is turned off. Arterial signal shown returning from sample volume ahead of venous echo. **C**, Crystal is activated to receive signal returning from sample volume. **D**, Crystal is turned off until next signal is sent; signals returned are not received.

ner) to allow precise placement of the sample volume. This is accomplished by moving the cursor, or ***sample volume,*** on the B-mode imaging screen to the site at which Doppler insonation is to occur.

The ***spectral waveform*** provides the most complete form of Doppler output (Fig. 3-4). Waveform output can be on paper, a display screen, or both. Multiple frequencies of the signal are processed simul-

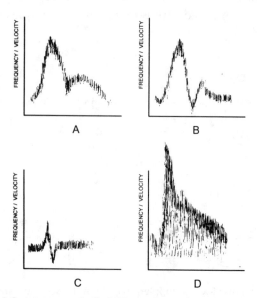

Fig. 3-4. Spectrum analysis. **A,** Normal waveform, low resistance. **B,** Normal waveform, moderate resistance. **C,** High resistance waveform caused by distal obstruction. **D,** High peak systolic velocity, broad spectrum waveform caused by tight stenosis.

taneously, with the intensity on the display proportional to the number of reflectors moving at a given velocity. High peak systolic frequency signals indicate the presence of a stenosis at the site of insonation. Low velocities indicate reduced flow, suggesting the presence of a proximal or distal flow obstruction. "Broadening" of the spectrum—the display of a wide range of velocities or frequencies—indicates turbulence, whereas a "narrow" spectrum of frequencies suggests laminar flow. Forward flow in diastole suggests low resistance, while low flow or no diastolic flow (with or without flow reversal) suggests a high outflow resistance.

Although the Doppler accurately measures changes in frequency, the clinician is more interested in the *velocity* of the blood flow. The velocity of the moving blood is related to the frequency shift of the returning echoes by the Doppler equation:

$$\text{Velocity of blood} = \frac{\text{Frequency shift} \times \text{Speed of sound in tissue}}{2 \times \text{Operating frequency} \times \text{Cos } \theta}$$

Thus, to determine the blood flow velocity, the *angle* (θ) between the Doppler signal and the *direction* of blood flow must be known (Fig. 3-5). Therefore the angle of the ultrasound beam to the vessel being insonated must be accurately measured. The combination of a B-mode ultrasound imager and the Doppler flow detector in the duplex scanner makes this possible. While the scanner can accurately measure flow velocity,

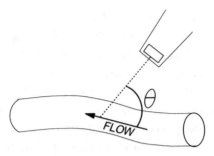

Fig. 3-5. Doppler angle is the angle between the direction of blood flow and the ultrasound beam. The angle is used in the Doppler equation to convert the measured frequency shift to blood flow velocity.

the determination of volume flow is less accurate and more difficult, since it requires measurement of both lumen area and average flow velocity over the whole cardiac cycle.

Magnetic resonance flowmeter. The magnetic resonance (MR) flowmeter is a relatively new device for arterial flow measurement and must be differentiated from standard MR imagers. It is a small unit designed to measure blood flow only and does not provide a high-resolution, useful image. Claims have been made as to its ability to replace plethysmographic techniques and to provide accurate flow information previously not attainable. Experience with this device is limited at present, and recommendations regarding its use cannot be made.

IMAGING

B-mode scan. The B-mode, or brightness-mode, ultrasound imager displays a two-dimensional image based on the reflection of sound waves at tissue interfaces, where changes in density exist. The duration of time for return of the ultrasound signal and its strength are reflected in the image by the distance of the object from its interface and its brightness, respectively. A multitude of images (each represented by a dot on the screen) are produced by an array of piezoelectric crystals in the transducer and combine to produce a two-dimensional picture, or B-mode scan image.

The B-scan is capable of producing an image of the blood vessel walls as well as of intraluminal densities. Thus vessel diameter, intraluminal plaque, thrombus, and intimal flaps can be evaluated. The B-scan can also identify pseudoaneurysms, hematomas, other fluid collections, and masses. Although the B-mode scan picture is usually able to produce an image of vessels, it *cannot* give information regarding the blood flow through a vessel. Indeed, it cannot reliably be used to determine patency or the extent of stenosis of a vessel—information most readily obtained with the use of the Doppler signal.

A *duplex scanner* is an ultrasound device that *integrates* the B-mode scan and the pulsed Doppler flow detector. A recent innovation in the duplex scanner has been the addition of color to the ultrasound B-mode image to display blood flow. *Color Doppler imaging* is accomplished by evaluation of pulsed-wave Doppler signals throughout an area of the image. The mean Doppler velocity determined at each point or *pixel* on the B-mode display is converted to a color. By convention, red is designated to represent flow *toward* the scanning probe and blue *away* from the probe. Velocity differences within the vessel are represented by variations of the brightness of the displayed colors. The color Doppler display has allowed rapid identification of vessels and grafts. Likewise, stenotic areas are readily identified as regions of increased or turbulent flow and are highlighted with bright colors. Color Doppler, however, *does not* reduce the importance of spectral analysis, since it does not provide the same detailed flow assessment. The technician must still insonate specific sites in the vessel to produce the spectral waveform.

CT scan. Computed tomography (CT) is the radiographic technique of reconstructing a cross-sectional image based on the information obtained from a series of narrow X-ray beams passing at different angles through the section under study. Newer techniques, such as spiral scanning, allow more rapid acquisition of images, with improved quality. While "noncontrast" CT scans can image blood vessels, CT images are significantly enhanced by the intravascular injection of contrast material; however, this increases the invasiveness of the procedure.

Magnetic resonance imaging. Although the technique of nuclear magnetic resonance analysis has been available since the late 1940s, it was not until the early 1980s that the technique became clinically available. Magnetic resonance imaging (MRI) is a noninvasive method that relies on the interaction of hydrogen nuclei, which are subjected to a strong magnetic field, and radiowaves.

Magnetic resonance angiography (MRA) techniques enable the imaging of blood moving through tissues. Laminar flow is more easily imaged than turbulent flow because of more stable movement of the molecules maintaining their alignment in the magnetic field. Turbulent flow produces a more random movement of blood molecules, thereby preventing proper alignment. Therefore a stenotic area with turbulent flow will be displayed as an absence of flow and can be misinterpreted as an occlusion of the vessel. Under ideal conditions, however, MRA techniques can provide high-resolution imaging of vessels as small as 2 mm in diameter.

Application of Noninvasive Tests

EXTREMITY SEGMENTAL PRESSURE MEASUREMENT. Segmental pressure measurements of the lower extremity are typically taken at the thigh, calf, and ankle levels, and in the great toe when distal disease is suspected (Fig. 3-6). This examination is indicated for the evaluation of peripheral arterial disease and should be included in the assessment of ischemic symptoms or lesions of the extremities. Segmental pressure measurements are also useful in the evaluation of a therapeutic procedure (bypass or angioplasty) to obtain an objective measurement of its effect. Not only is the direct pressure measurement at each level important, but also the comparison of each measurement with the brachial pressure is commonly used. Thus the *index* of the level being evaluated is calculated by dividing the pressure measured by the brachial pressure. The ***ankle-brachial index*** (ABI), the most commonly used of the indices, is calculated by dividing the systolic blood pressure at the ankle by the brachial systolic blood pressure.

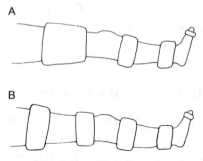

Fig. 3-6. Segmental pressure cuff placement: thigh, calf, ankle, and great toe. **A,** Thigh one-cuff technique. **B,** Thigh two-cuff technique.

Thigh pressure. Thigh pressure measurements are made with either the one-cuff or two-cuff technique (see Fig. 3-6). A single long 18 cm cuff is used for the one-cuff method; the two-cuff technique uses small 10 to 12 cm cuffs, placed on the upper thigh and at the above-the-knee position. It is generally thought that the two-cuff method better differentiates superficial femoral from aortoiliac disease. Since the upper cuff is less likely to be affected by superficial femoral disease, a low reading is more specific for aortoiliac disease. The normal pressure at the thigh should be greater than the brachial arterial pressure. When the thigh pressure of the upper cuff is the same or less than brachial pressure (index ≤ 1.0), a significant aortoiliac stenosis is likely to be present. However, false positive results occur when a common or deep femoral artery occlusion or stenosis is present. Accordingly, interpretations of thigh pressures should also be based on the quality of the femoral pulse or femoral artery pressures. While false negative readings do occur, especially in a patient with a large thigh, the finding of an index >1.2 is fairly reliable for ruling out significant aortoiliac disease.

Pressure gradients. In the absence of a significant degree of arterial obstruction, the difference in pressure between any two levels in the leg should not exceed 20 to 30 mm Hg. Likewise, when the two legs are compared at the same level, a greater than 20 mm Hg gradient is also consistent with a significant proximal stenosis on the side with the lower pressure. In general, all normal levels should have an index (ratio to the brachial pressure) of >1.0.

Ankle pressures. The ankle pressure measurement and the *ankle-brachial index* (ABI) are reliable, and widely used, parameters for the assessment of lower extremity occlusive disease. As with the other levels, an index of <1.0 is consistent with significant proximal disease. The ABI does not always correlate well with clinical symptoms, although certain guidelines have been defined. Mild and moderately severe claudication is usually associated with an ABI from 0.5 to 1.0, while severe claudication and advanced ischemia are usually found only with an ABI of <0.5.

Toe pressures. Toe pressures are measured when calcified arteries are present and when there is concern about distal disease, especially in the presence of ischemic lesions. Measurements are performed using a small toe cuff and either a strain-gauge plethysmograph or a photoplethysmograph to detect the pulsations in the tip of the toe. These measurements are particularly useful when calf and ankle pressures are falsely elevated as a result of medial calcification. Arteries of the toe are usually less affected by calcifications; thus toe pressure measurements remain reliable. Normal toe pressures are about half of the ankle pressures and are usually over 50 mm Hg. Pressures of less than 50 mm Hg indicate significant disease, consistent with claudication and ischemic lesions. When pressures are below 30 mm Hg, disease is severe and revascularization is usually required to obtain healing.

EXTREMITY SEGMENTAL ARTERIAL PLETHYSMOGRAPHY. Segmental air plethysmography is performed for the same indications as segmental pressure measurements. Evaluation of the plethysmographic waveform is based on the shape of the curve and its amplitude (Fig. 3-7). Early disease is characterized by loss of the dicrotic notch, but a more rounded peak signifies moderate disease. Severe disease is associated with a flattened waveform and a slow upstroke and downstroke. Amplitude measurements in the presence of minimal to moderate degrees of disease are quite variable from patient to patient, because they are influenced by cardiac stroke volume, blood pressure, blood volume, vasomotor tone, and the size of the limb. However,

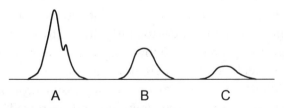

Fig. 3-7. Air plethysmography arterial waveforms. **A**, Normal. **B**, Moderate disease—rounded peak and loss of dicrotic notch. **C**, Severe disease—slow upstroke and downstroke, low amplitude.

very low amplitude measurements—those with <5 mm chart deflection—are consistently associated with severe, usually multisegmental, disease. When followed over time by a consistent technique, amplitude is a reliable means for evaluating progression of occlusive disease.

Thigh plethysmography has been shown to generally underestimate the severity of aortoiliac disease, and as with segmental pressures, disease in the superficial femoral artery cannot always be differentiated from more proximal disease. Normally amplitudes in the calf are 25% greater than those in the thigh. If this increase, also known as *augmentation,* is not present, superficial femoral or popliteal artery stenosis is likely. Air plethysmography of the lower extremity is most accurate when disease involves only one level, with increasing accuracy at the more distal levels.

STRESS TESTING
Exercise testing. It is possible that the severity of occlusive disease may be such that the reduction in *resting* blood flow rate is too insignificant to affect the segmental pressure or plethysmographic measurements. At higher blood flow rates, however, a stenosis that is insignificant at rest may produce a pressure drop as a result of the increased flow rate and decreased peheral resistance. This is the rationale for the *exercise stress test.* Exercise increases the demand for oxygen,

thereby dilating arterioles and lowering their resistance to flow. This in turn will increase the blood flow to the distal vascular bed and produce a pressure gradient across a proximal stenosis. An exercise-induced pressure drop will occur in the calf in the presence of most superficial femoral artery stenoses. The stress test is also a valuable measure for assessing a patient's exercise tolerance. The typical protocol involves treadmill walking for 5 minutes at 2 mph on a 10% grade. Arm and ankle pressures are measured before testing, immediately upon completion of the walk, and then at 30-second intervals for several minutes. A drop in ankle pressure of 20 mm Hg below brachial pressure indicates a significant degree of stenosis. More severe disease is associated with a greater drop in ankle pressure and a delayed return of pressure to the baseline.

Reactive hyperemia. Reactive hyperemia testing is an alternative method for increasing blood flow across a presumed stenosis that has not been identified by resting pressure measurements. Inflation of a thigh cuff occludes arterial inflow to the foot, thereby producing ischemia of the calf and foot. The cuff is then released, resulting in a transient increase in blood flow over the baseline, thus unmasking a stenosis not appreciated with standard testing protocols. Hyperemia stress testing is useful if a patient is unable to ambulate or a treadmill is not available. Exercise testing, however, is more reliable, and is the preferred technique.

CAROTID AND VERTEBRAL ARTERY DUPLEX SCAN.
The duplex scan is the mainstay of the noninvasive
diagnosis of carotid arterial disease. It is indicated when
an internal carotid artery stenosis is suspected on the
basis of the history (neurologic symptoms referable to
the cerebral circulation) or physical examination (carotid bruit or pulsatile neck mass). Although a simple
Doppler instrument can detect a stenosis, the imaging
and accurate placement of the Doppler sample volume provides a higher degree of reliability. Criteria
outlined by Strandness based on spectrum analysis
are used to categorize carotid artery stenosis and have
been demonstrated to be highly accurate (Table 3-1).

Occlusion of the internal carotid artery (ICA) can
also be detected using the duplex scan. This requires
careful examination of the carotid bulb to ensure that
a small channel with high velocity flow is not present.
The presence of a high-resistance waveform in the

Table 3-1. Duplex Criteria for Internal Carotid
Artery Stenosis

Stenosis (%)	Peak Systolic Velocity (cm/sec)	Peak Diastolic Velocity (cm/sec)	Waveform
15-49	<125	<140	Broadened
50-79	>125	<140	Broadened
>80	>125	>140	Broadened

Based on data from Strandness DE. Duplex Scanning in Vascular Disorders. New York: Raven Press, 1990.

common carotid artery should alert the examiner to the possibility of an ICA occlusion.

Classification of atherosclerotic plaque in the carotid bulb is also available from the duplex scan examination. Identification of calcifications and the differentiation between homogenous and heterogeneous plaque have been clinically valuable pieces of information. Attempts at further classification, such as the detection of intraplaque hemorrhage or ulceration, have *not* been found to be reliable or able to predict clinical events accurately.

The cerebrovascular duplex scan should include the assessment of the vertebral vessels. These are located posterior to the carotid arteries and usually cannot be completely visualized because of their location in the cervical vertebrae. The duplex scan is reliable in detecting a significant stenosis at the origin of the vessel from the subclavian artery. Detection of vertebral artery flow reversal may also be evaluated and indicates disease of the more proximal subclavian/innominate vessels. This information is useful in the evaluation for the subclavian steal syndrome.

TRANSCRANIAL DOPPLER IMAGING. Transcranial Doppler imaging is a reliable method for providing information about the intracranial vessels—primarily those of the circle of Willis. Generally, clinical application has been limited to identification of vasospasm following subarachnoid hemorrhage and detection of intracranial stenosis and AV malformations. An additional use has been continuous monitoring of intracranial blood flow during carotid endarterectomy or cardiopulmonary bypass. The transcranial Doppler technique is performed "blindly" with placement of the signal based on anatomic location, and assessment of the returning signal information confirming the direction and configuration of the imaged vessel. The normal transcranial Doppler flow velocity as measured in the middle cerebral artery is greater than 45 cm/sec and in the anterior and posterior cerebral arteries it is greater than 35 cm/sec. A reduction in middle cerebral flow velocity of up to 65% during internal carotid artery cross-clamping is consistent with adequate cerebral perfusion.

PERIPHERAL ARTERIAL DUPLEX SCAN. Duplex scan assessment of peripheral arteries has been limited to the assessment of aneurysms of the femoral and popliteal arteries and assessment of stenotic lesions for which transluminal angioplasty is considered. The duplex scanner is a highly accurate tool for diagnosing aneurysmal disease. Diameter measurement is more accurate than arteriography, since the *outer* edge of the vessel wall and the extent of mural thrombus is well defined using B-mode imaging. The identification of pseudoaneurysms is aided by the use of color Doppler imaging, which clearly displays the flow from artery into the pseudoaneurysm cavity.

The comparison of duplex scanning with arteriography of lower extremity vessels has shown it to be accurate for the identification of stenoses greater than 50%. Specificity of identifying lesions of the iliac, femoral and popliteal vessels is greater than 90%, while sensitivity of the same vessels is between 70% and 90%. Although the general evaluation of the vasculature is not practical using the duplex scan, evaluation of specific areas can be useful. A patient with a suspected superficial femoral artery stenosis and claudication may undergo duplex scanning to identify a lesion that would be amenable to angioplasty *before* the patient is subjected to angiography. The finding of a short stenosis may lead one to recommend angioplasty, whereas a long occlusion, known to have a lower success rate with angioplasty, may lead one to recommend against balloon dilatation.

BYPASS GRAFT SURVEILLANCE. Evaluation and monitoring of bypass grafts, especially in the lower extremity, are commonly performed with the duplex scan, plethysmography, and pressure measurements. Similar to the evaluation of native vessels, stenoses are identified with the duplex scan by elevations in peak systolic velocity, usually greater than 250 cm/sec. High grade stenoses are associated with reduced velocity in the remainder of the graft distal to the graft stenosis. Thus, a peak systolic velocity *less* than 45 cm/sec in a vein graft is usually, although not always, associated with a significant stenosis that requires correction. When low velocity is found, the graft must be insonated completely to find the area of stenosis. Duplex scans of a bypass should be carried out at routine intervals. The initial scan is usually performed within the first 30 days, followed by a repeat scan at least every 3 months for the first year and every 6 months thereafter. The finding of an increased velocity without the presence of a high grade lesion requiring correction is an indication to repeat the scan at more frequent intervals.

Bypass graft monitoring is also assisted by the use of plethysmography and pressure measurements. While in the immediate postoperative period there may not be an improvement of the pressure or amplitude, within 48 hours an increase of at least 0.15 in the ABI should be demonstrable. A subsequent drop of that same amount, or a decrease in the air plethysmography amplitude by 5 mm, suggests compromise of the graft and indicates the need for further investigation—either by duplex scan or arteriography.

DUPLEX SCAN OF AORTA/BRANCHES. Duplex ultrasonography of the abdominal aorta is commonly performed for the assessment of aortic size. B-scan imaging of the abdominal aorta is accurate and highly reliable in the diagnosis of an infrarenal *abdominal aortic aneurysm* (AAA). The diameter measurements are as accurate as those with the CT scan, and it is a more practical modality for following the size of an aneurysm over time. The use of the duplex scan for evaluation of a potentially ruptured AAA is generally *not* recommended. Emergency evaluation of the acute, unprepared abdomen is usually suboptimal and may delay the use of more definitive studies.

The lumen of the aorta and iliac arteries can also be evaluated with the duplex scan to search for a source of distal emboli. The detection of irregular plaque on the aortic wall may suggest an embolic source. Evaluation of the suprarenal AAA is best performed with a CT scan, because the accuracy of Duplex scanning at this level is suboptimal.

The diagnosis of **renal artery stenosis** utilizing the duplex scan has been well documented. However, difficulties may exist in insonating the renal arteries because of their depth. An increase in the peak systolic velocity to >3.5 times the aortic peak velocity is consistent with a significant stenosis (>60%). This has been shown to be highly specific (97%) and strongly correlated with renal arteriography (r = 0.93). Positive results of a renal artery duplex evaluation indicate the need for arteriography.

The **celiac** and **superior mesenteric arteries** can also be assessed for areas of stenosis. However, the ability to quantify disease is less well established in these vessels because of the extent of collateralization of mesenteric blood flow. Flow through the mesenteric vessels is highly variable, exhibiting a high-resistance spectral waveform in the fasting state and a postprandial low-resistance waveform. Chronic mesenteric ischemia presents with stenosis or occlusion in *both* the superior mesenteric and celiac arteries. Duplex ultrasonography has not been useful in the diagnosis of acute mesenteric ischemia because of the difficulties in scanning the acute abdomen.

MAGNETIC RESONANCE IMAGING: ABDOMINAL VASCULATURE. Imaging of all structures in the abdomen and retroperitoneum, including the large vessels, is effectively carried out with magnetic resonance imaging. Indications are similar to those for the CT scan, namely, the identification of aneurysmal disease. MRI is also useful for the identification of vena caval and iliac vein thrombosis. It is *not* advised for the identification of a "leaking" or potentially ruptured AAA, since monitoring of the patient is limited during the examination.

MAGNETIC RESONANCE ANGIOGRAPHY

Cerebrovascular. MRA can visualize the arch vessels as well as the cervical and intracranial vasculature. High-grade stenoses are not reliably differentiated from occlusions, and therefore the scan has yielded suboptimal results in evaluation of a diseased carotid artery bifurcation. It is frequently used, however, to *confirm* the finding of a high-grade carotid stenosis on duplex scan, thus obviating the need for cerebral contrast angiography.

Peripheral arteries. Currently MRA is not used for the assessment of extremity vessels because of its difficulties with imaging high-grade stenoses. Although several institutions have advocated its use in replacing peripheral angiography, the computer software required for the detailed high-resolution imaging is *not* universally available. Therefore this technology remains confined to a few specialized centers with a particular interest in this field.

Aorta and its branches. MRA is useful for the imaging of normal and aneurysmal vessels of the abdomen. The relationship of an AAA to surrounding vascular structures (renal veins and arteries and mesenteric arteries) has been extremely useful. Aortoiliac occlusive disease is not readily evaluated because of the difficulties with the imaging of high grade stenoses, as noted above.

VENOUS DUPLEX SCAN

Thrombosis. Duplex ultrasonography reliably detects thrombosis in peripheral veins. The technique used involves imaging the vein on the B-mode scan followed by cross sectional compression of the vessel with the scan probe. In the absence of thrombus, this should cause a flattening of the vein, with apposition of the anterior and posterior walls (Fig. 3-8). If the vein cannot be fully compressed, it is likely because of the presence of intraluminal thrombus. The absence of flow is confirmed with Doppler spectral analysis. This

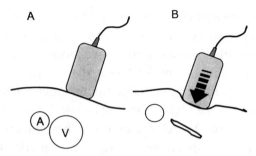

Fig. 3-8. Duplex scan detection of venous thrombosis. **A,** The vessels are first visualized in cross section to identify the artery and vein. **B,** The transducer is then used to apply compression to the vein. Complete apposition of its walls indicates no thrombus is present.

maneuver is reliable for the detection of thrombus in all major accessible veins of the lower and upper extremities with high levels of agreement with venography. The chronicity of a thrombus may be inferred by its heterogenicity and the presence of detectable collateral veins.

The duplex scan has replaced contrast venography as the gold standard for the diagnosis of deep venous thrombosis. Venography is now used only for cases in which ultrasound yields inconclusive findings. *Impedance plethysmography* can accurately identify outflow occlusion of the leg but does not detect *partially* occlusive thrombus.

Reflux. Chronic venous insufficiency is caused by valvular reflux or incompetence of the deep and perforating veins of the lower extremity. Duplex ultrasonography has been used to detect these incompetent valves and to determine the appropriateness of various therapies. Valvular evaluation requires the identification of a valve followed by maneuvers (Valsalva or manual compression) to observe closure of or reflux past the identified valve. The use of pneumatic cuffs that can be rapidly inflated is recommended to produce sufficient reverse venous flow to force closure of the valves. If manual compression is used, an insufficient amount of reversed flow can occur and a false positive result could be obtained. Ideally, the valve at the saphenofemoral junction, valves in the femoral and popliteal veins, and perforating veins in the calf and thigh should be identified and evaluated. A normal valve, when subjected to sufficient reversed flow, should close within 1 second, and most close in less than 0.5 seconds.

VENOUS REFLUX PLETHYSMOGRAPHY. Physiologic assessment of venous insufficiency can be performed using plethysmographic techniques. The presence and severity of venous reflux is evaluated at a time at which muscular contractions should be returning blood to the heart. The photoplethysmograph has been shown to be reliable in evaluating deep venous reflux when the perforating valves are incompetent. The test is performed by placing the PPG probe on the skin and having the patient tip-toe five times in succession to cause strong calf contractions. The tracing should show a drop in skin blood congestion during the contractions, followed, at rest, by a slow return to the baseline in 30 seconds or greater (Fig. 3-9). If recovery to baseline occurs in less than 20 seconds, significant reflux is present. When severe reflux is present, there is only a minimal drop in venous congestion with exercise, and

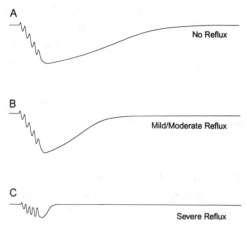

Fig. 3-9. Venous reflux photoplethysmography. A, In the normal limb a series of calf contractions will cause marked lowering of the signal, followed by a slow return to baseline. B, With moderate reflux, the signal will return to baseline quicker. C, In the limb with severe reflux, there is a minimal reduction in the signal level, followed by a rapid return to baseline.

a rapid return to the baseline. The test is usually repeated with a tourniquet in place on the thigh. This occludes the superficial venous system and eliminates its influence on total reflux. The presence of competent perforating veins will prevent the accurate assessment of the deep vein system using PPG.

Recently an alternative method using a large cuff air plethysmograph has been reported. In this technique a large cuff is placed on the calf after it is carefully measured to determine the volume of tissue under the calf. With this method one can determine the actual volume of fluid removed from the leg with each calf contraction and can establish a ***venous ejection fraction.*** This technique does *not* depend on the incompetence of the perforating system to assess the deep veins accurately.

DUPLEX VEIN MAPPING. The preoperative assessment of veins available for bypass grafting remains a concern for surgeons. Venography has been used in cases in which the native ipsilateral greater saphenous vein was previously used or when disease of the vein was suspected. The use of the in situ vein bypass has led to the use of the duplex scanner to image the superficial venous system. The evaluation involves imaging superficial layers of the leg, and the application of compression maneuvers on the vein to confirm patency. Measurements of the vein diameter are also carried out, although there is considerable underestimation of the size the vein will achieve when subjected to arterial pressure. Vein mapping is most useful in the patient undergoing secondary procedures in which vein patency is questioned, or when arm vein must be used. However, the accuracy of vein mapping remains somewhat imperfect, with occasional false positive and false negative results.

BIBLIOGRAPHY

Baker JD. The vascular laboratory. In Moore WS, ed. Vascular Surgery: A Comprehensive Review. Philadelphia: WB Saunders, 1991, pp 168-185.

Strandness DE. Duplex Scanning in Vascular Disorders. New York: Raven Press, 1990.

Sumner DS. Noninvasive assessment of peripheral arterial occlusive disease. In Rutherford RB, ed. Vascular Surgery. Philadelphia: WB Saunders, 1989, pp 61-111.

Sumner DS. Objective diagnostic techniques: Role of vascular lab. In Rutherford RB, ed. Vascular Surgery. Philadelphia: WB Saunders, 1989, pp 41-60.

4

Angiography and Other Catheter-Directed Techniques

Michael B. Silva, Jr. • *Charles D. Franco*

Arteriography

In the evaluation of patients with peripheral vascular disease, a detailed history and attentive physical examination can often determine the level of atherosclerotic occlusive lesions and estimate its severity. Noninvasive vascular studies should be used to substantiate the clinical impression. Arteriography, an invasive procedure with inherent risks, is rarely used as a primary method of diagnosis and should be obtained only after a decision has been made to intervene. Arteriography provides a detailed image of current arterial anatomy, allowing the clinician to select the most appropriate therapeutic alternative. Therapy may be surgical or "minimally invasive" utilizing one of the endovascular techniques such as percutaneous transluminal angioplasty or atherectomy, alone or in conjunction with thrombolytic therapy.

DEFINITION AND FACTORS INFLUENCING QUALITY. Arteriography involves displacement of flowing blood in an artery by radiopaque material during roentgenographic exposure of the area in which the artery lies. The quality of an arteriogram, and its utility, is dependent on numerous factors. The experienced angiographer must choose the most appropriate contrast agent, select the best radiographic projection, obtain access into the desired portion of the arterial system, select the appropriate injection volume and correct rate of injection, synchronizing with rapid filming machinery in an effort to visualize the area in question. Compromise of any one of these factors can, at a minimum, affect the quality and usefulness of an angiogram, and, in the extreme, place the patient at risk for serious complications.

NEEDLE TECHNIQUES AND APPROACHES FOR ACCESS. In the earliest method of arteriography, contrast material was injected directly through a needle placed into an artery. This has largely been replaced by catheter systems using radiolucent plastic sheaths with soft flexible tips, posing less risk of intimal dissection or injury. Either the catheter-over-needle technique or the Seldinger method, using a wire guidance system, can be successfully employed.

There are four basic approaches for obtaining access to the arterial system: transfemoral, translumbar, transaxillary and brachial. The area to be demonstrated, in combination with each patient's distribution of disease, dictates the specific approach chosen. The femoral approach is generally suitable for demonstration of the carotid arteries, upper extremity vessels, the aorta and its abdominal visceral branches, and the infrainguinal peripheral arterial system. If aortoiliac or local disease precludes passage of a wire or catheter from the femoral artery, a transaxillary, or (less commonly) a translumbar approach can be used. The brachial artery may also be used as an alternative approach and may be preferred by some for selective coronary artery catheterization.

Regardless of the approach, a number of catheters with curves, slants, hooks, and even steerable guidewires are now available. When they are used by an experienced angiographer, access into almost any vessel can be obtained. The development of these highly selective catheterization techniques has facilitated advances in alternative intra-arterial therapies, including infusion of thrombolytic, or other pharmacologic, agents and transcatheter embolization techniques.

Contrast Venography

In the diagnosis of venous pathologic conditions, contrast venography has been the standard against which all other techniques have been evaluated. When properly performed, it is highly sensitive and specific for the presence of venous clots in all of the major veins of the leg, abdomen, and arm. In contrast to arteriography, however, venography is more difficult to perform and the resulting studies are less easily interpreted. The studies can be costly, time-consuming, and painful. Additionally a small number of patients (less than 5%) will develop thrombophlebitis as a direct result of the contrast medium itself. These factors have prompted clinicians to utilize noninvasive tests as the initial diagnostic method in patients in whom deep venous thrombosis is suspected.

The duplex scan has provided an attractive alternative to contrast venography. It is a direct, noninvasive examination that is painless and risk free. It can be accomplished relatively quickly at the bedside, with repeat examinations performed as necessary. When performed by an experienced technologist, the accuracy of duplex scanning for detection of deep vein thrombosis in the major segmental axial veins has been shown to be comparable with that of contrast venography.

Interventional Angiography

Interventional angiography is a growing field that encompasses a number of technical applications of catheters and specific devices designed to be a primary therapeutic modality in the treatment of arteriosclerosis obliterans. Percutaneous transluminal angioplasty, stents, atherectomy, and the judicious use of thrombolytic therapy are now commonly employed treatment modalities. These procedures do not supplant surgery but rather, when appropriately utilized, complement and expand the available therapeutic armamentarium.

Percutaneous Transluminal Angioplasty (PTA)

The PTA catheter is designed with an inflatable, nondeformable balloon at the distal end. When inflated, the balloon cracks the constricting atherosclerotic plaque and stretches the underlying media to enlarge the lumen. The smooth muscle of the media, as well as elastin and collagen fibers, are damaged in the process. The injured vessel wall is expected to heal in its newly expanded posture, resulting in a larger lumen.

PTA has been used with varying success to treat lesions in the aortic, iliac, femoral, popliteal, mesenteric, and renal circulations. The best results have been obtained in the iliac arteries, and these results may be improved by the addition of expandable metal stents. The ideal lesion is a short (less than 2 cm), hemodynamically significant stenosis in an otherwise relatively normal artery. Under these circumstances, initial success rates can be expected to be as high as 95%, with reported 5-year patency rates of 75% to 90%.

PTA of femoropopliteal lesions has had neither the initial success rate nor the long-term patency seen in iliac artery angioplasty. The numbers range widely, but given a select group of patients with the most favorable lesions (short stenoses in otherwise normal arteries), initial success can be achieved in approximately 85% of patients, with long-term patency approaching 70%. In arteries with more diffuse disease or longer segments of stenosis, long-term patency is usually limited to a matter of months.

Atherectomy

There are currently four FDA-approved atherectomy devices available for clinical use: the Simpson Atherocath, the Kensey atherectomy device, the Auth Rotablator and the transluminal extraction catheter. Each has a different mechanism of operation, but all attempt to selectively shave and remove atheromatous debris from atherosclerotic diseased arteries. To date none of these devices have improved upon the restenosis rate of conventional balloon angioplasty. It has been hypothesized that the intimal injury created by necessity with these instruments induces a myointimal hyperplastic response which eventually compromises expected results.

Thrombolytic Therapy

Thrombolytic therapy can be employed as a primary treatment modality for embolic or thrombotic events. Alternatively, it can be used as an adjunctive procedure to identify the underlying source of an arterial occlusion and enable the clinician to select the most appropriate treatment option. Thrombolytic agents in use include streptokinase, urokinase and tissue plasminogen activator. Streptokinase and urokinase are exogenous plasminogen activators that produce fibrinolysis by activating the body's natural fibrinolytic system. Specifically, they mediate conversion of plasminogen to plasmin which in turn lyses fibrin clots.

Streptokinase is a product of streptococci and, as a foreign protein, is antigenic. Allergic reactions and poor patient tolerance are not uncommon. Urokinase (UK) has been isolated from human urine and cultured from embryonic kidney cells. It has a half-life of approximately 14 minutes. It is nonantigenic and its pyrogenicity is low. Recombinant DNA technology has been used to make a recombinant urokinase. Clinical trials are under way to affirm its clinical equivalence to the tissue culture urokinase. Tissue plasminogen activator is also a product of recombinant DNA technology. Although it is a poor activator of the fibrinolytic system in the absence of fibrin, its high affinity for plasminogen in the presence of fibrin allows efficient lysis of the fibrin clot without significant conversion of plasminogen in circulating plasma.

For intra-arterial therapy the usual technique for delivery of thrombolytic agents involves the placement of an indwelling arterial catheter into the thrombus. High doses of a lytic agent (for example, 250,000

U/hr of UK) are infused for 2 to 4 hours, followed by repeat transcatheter arteriography. The infusion catheter is advanced as warranted, and lower doses of the lytic agent are infused for prolonged periods of time; interval angiography is performed to assess the efficacy of treatment. Throughout the process the patient must be continuously monitored in an appropriate setting, with periodic hematologic evaluation for assessment of the level of systemic fibrinolysis.

Other Endovascular Techniques

The use of intra-arterial stents is currently under investigation as an alternative or adjunct to angioplasty. Similarly, laser-tipped devices have been evaluated as a method of increasing the number of atherosclerotic lesions which are amenable to balloon dilatation. Theoretically, the laser is used to facilitate the creation of a lumen that is otherwise inaccessible using standard guidewire techniques. In practice, results to date have not been encouraging, and the development of new guidewires has made the laser-tipped device almost obsolete. Endovascular procedures are more commonly being applied at the extremes of the clinical spectrum, where arterial surgery either would not be traditionally justifiable (as in the claudicator with a discrete stenosis) or could not be tolerated, because of excessive operative risk. However, the recent introduction of endoluminal stented grafts has the potential to significantly alter the future practice of vascular surgery.

The development of interventional angiography has required a cooperative effort between vascular surgeons and angiographers. These patients must be evaluated and cared for as if they were to undergo a significant operative procedure. Angiographic interventional techniques are technically demanding and should be performed in a setting where sufficient support personnel are available to care for the patients and handle any complications that may arise.

Complications

Most complications can be divided into one of two groups: those associated with the administration of contrast material and those related to mechanical injury to the vascular system from manipulation of the catheter or from management of the puncture site.

Contrast media. Contrast media are toxic substances. The toxicity is a result of their hypertonicity and intrinsic chemotoxicity. New lower osmolar contrast substances are available that are nonionic and have been shown to have less toxicity. These benefits have not yet been proven conclusively in human subjects, but these agents are better tolerated, with less pain than usually accompanies the use of conventional ionic contrast material. The newer agents are being used selectively rather than routinely in most centers, however, because of their significantly added expense.

Allergic reactions. The overall incidence of allergic reactions in studies using contrast media is approximately 5%. The risk of fatal reaction with administration of a conventional contrast medium is between 1 in 16,000 and 1 in 117,000. The likelihood of a fatal reaction with the low-osmolar media may be somewhat lower.

Nephrotoxicity. Contrast media induce a diuresis secondary to their increased osmolarity. The mechanism of contrast-induced renal damage is not completely understood but is known to be related to the dose and concentration of the agent and the duration of exposure. Patients with low renal blood flow, preexisting renal insufficiency, diabetes mellitus, proteinuria, and dehydration are at an increased risk of contrast-induced renal failure. Preangiographic dehydration appears to be the most important negative factor in the development of a postangiographic decline in renal function.

Cardiopulmonary toxicity. Contrast media are vasodilators, and the standard higher osmotic type is known to be a direct myocardial depressant. The resultant hypotension can have serious consequences in patients with ischemic myocardial or cerebrovascular disease. Also, patients with a pheochromocytoma may develop hypertensive crisis with contrast injection, and any patient may develop severe pulmonary edema.

Neurologic toxicity. Contrast media injected into the vascular system may induce alterations in the blood-brain barrier, with direct neurotoxicity, causing convulsions, paresis, cortical blindness, or frank stroke.

MECHANICAL COMPLICATIONS. Local catheter complications at the puncture site include bleeding, thrombosis, pseudoaneurysm, and formation of an arteriovenous fistula. The overall incidence of catheter-induced complications is 0.5% with a transfemoral route, 0.6% with a translumbar route, and 2.0% when using the transaxillary route. Bleeding is the most common complication of arterial catheterization and is usually noted within a short period after completion of the study, although it may go undetected because of the suprainguinal retroperitoneal location of the puncture site. If the arterial wall defect persists in its communication with the adjacent hematoma, a fibrous capsule will be formed, producing a pseudoaneurysm. Thrombosis, another major catheter-related complication, is related to the size of the artery being cannulated. Consequently the brachial artery approach has the highest incidence of postcannulation thrombotic complications. The sequelae of hematoma formation are frequently worse with the axillary artery than with the femoral artery. An occult axillary nerve sheath hematoma may cause irreparable neurologic injury if the diagnosis is missed. Attentive neurologic follow-up is the only way to avoid this disaster.

Preangiography Checklist

History and Physical Examination. Obtain and record accurate baseline data on the patient's complete vascular and neurologic examination so that appropriate post-procedure care can be rendered and complications can be quickly identified. Review aspects of the history pertinent to adverse contrast reactions or complications of catheterization:

    History of allergy or previous contrast reaction
    Renal failure
    Diabetes mellitus
    Recent myocardial infarction
    Hypertension
    Coagulopathy

Hydration. Hydration is one of the most critical preprocedure factors and can be easily accomplished. Intravenous fluids should be started and infused at a rate appropriate to the patient's overall fluid status. Diet can be clear liquids for the 8 hours before angioplasty. A patient should not be on NPO status unless an intravenous line is infusing appropriately.

Laboratory Data. Obtain baseline laboratory evaluation of renal function and coagulation profile including hemoglobin, hematocrit, and platelet count. For patients who will undergo thrombolytic therapy, additional baseline studies of the fibrinolytic system are indicated (fibrinogen and fibrin degradation products).

Informed Consent. Discuss the procedure, its risks, alternatives, and possible consequences with the patient. Obtain and record consent appropriately.

During cerebral angiography the added consequence of neurologic complications from mechanical factors is fortunately uncommon. The incidence of major complications (such as death, stroke, and access site problems requiring surgical intervention) has been reported to be approximately 0.16% in one large study. Transient ischemic attacks (TIAs) were reported to occur with a frequency of approximately 0.9% in another study.

The checklist on p. 72 provides guidelines for minimizing risks and reducing the potential for complications associated with the procedure.

BIBLIOGRAPHY

Ahn SS, Eton D, Moore WS. Endovascular surgery for peripheral arterial occlusive disease: A critical review. Ann Surg 216:3-16, 1992.

Berkowitz HD. Percutaneous arterial dilation for atherosclerotic lower extremity occlusive disease. In Ernst CB, Stanley JC, eds. Current Therapy in Vascular Surgery, 2nd ed. Philadelphia: BC Decker, 1991, pp 473-475.

Bourne EE, Kumpne DA. Percutaneous transluminal angioplasty and transcatheter embolization: Fundamental considerations. In Rutherford RB, ed. Vascular Surgery, 3rd ed. Philadelphia: WB Saunders, 1989, pp 328-341.

Johnston KW. Percutaneous arterial dilation for atherosclerotic aorto-iliac occlusive disease. In Ernst CB, Stanley JC, eds. Current Therapy in Vascular Surgery, 2nd ed. Philadelphia: BC Decker, 1991, pp 402-405.

Maddison FE, Kumpe DA, Rutherford RB, Redmond PL. Contrast arteriography. In Rutherford RB, ed. Vascular Surgery, 3rd ed. Philadelphia: WB Saunders, 1989, pp 157-177.

Redmond PL, Kilcoyne RF, Rose JS. Principles of angiography. In Rutherford RB, ed. Vascular Surgery, 3rd ed. Philadelphia: WB Saunders, 1989, pp 143-157.

5
Medical Evaluation of the Patient With Vascular Disease

William D. Suggs

Patients with peripheral vascular disease generally have multiple medical problems as a result of atherosclerotic involvement of their entire cardiovascular system. To define each patient's surgical risk and to maximize his or her medical condition before surgery, a thorough preoperative medical evaluation is essential to assess the extent and severity of each patient's medical disease.

Cardiac Evaluation

Patients with peripheral vascular disease often have concomitant coronary artery disease that must be evaluated before an operation is considered. Cardiac events account for 40% to 60% of early postoperative deaths in vascular patients. Forty percent of patients who have no history of cardiac disease and no electrocardiographic evidence of previous myocardial infarction will have at least one coronary artery with a hemodynamically significant lesion. Three-vessel disease or left main coronary artery disease may be present in up to 16% of these patients.

Careful history-taking should include screening for previous myocardial infarction, angina, or dyspnea on exertion. The dates and extent of any previous cardiac evaluation or revascularization should be recorded. Because of an inability to exercise, a vascular patient will often have coronary artery disease that is clinically silent. The cardiac workup can be structured by the indicators of cardiac disease. There are a variety of tests that can be used to evaluate the cardiac status of the patient.

Echocardiography and *radionuclide ventriculography* are used to assess the ventricular ejection fraction. It has been established that patients with an abnormal ejection fraction are more likely to have perioperative cardiac events, particularly those with an ejection fraction of less than 35%. However, many patients with a normal ejection fraction may have a significant degree of coronary artery disease. Therefore these tests are helpful in selecting the need for invasive monitoring but do not serve well as screening tests for coronary artery disease.

Exercise testing can be helpful in screening for patients who may need further cardiac evaluation. A positive test result is defined as one in which the heart rate reaches less than 85% of predicted value or one in which a patient experiences ST segment depression during exercise. The major limitation of this test is that most vascular patients have low exercise tolerance or may be medicated with beta-blockers or diuretics that limit the sensitivity of this test. Patients with a clearly positive test result should undergo cardiac catheterization before surgery.

The ***dipyridamole-thallium scan*** is an excellent screening test for the vascular patient. The dilatory effect of dipyridamole provides a physiologic substitute for exercise. Thallium is used to evaluate the cardiac perfusion. Dipyridamole is injected intravenously over a 4-minute period, followed by an injection of thallium-201. Isotope scans are obtained immediately after administration of thallium and again 4 hours later. Accurate interpretation of the scan requires comparison of the initial scan with the delayed images. Areas of viable myocardium are indicated by the prompt uptake of thallium. Areas with no thallium uptake ("fixed deficit") indicate previously infarcted myocardium. An area without uptake on initial scan but one in which isotope uptake is demonstrated on delayed images ("redistribution") represents an area of potentially ischemic myocardium. The presence of redistribution has proved to be a sensitive predictor of perioperative cardiac events. Patients with significant redistribution should be strongly considered for cardiac catheterization before surgery.

Cardiac catheterization is reserved for patients with a positive screening test to evaluate the need for cardiac revascularization before surgery. Patients who present with unstable or significant angina are also candidates for initial cardiac catheterization without undergoing screening tests.

Pulmonary Evaluation

Pulmonary assessment requires a thorough history and careful physical examination. The measurement of arterial blood gases and performance of pulmonary function tests are additional steps necessary for the adequate evaluation of respiratory function.

A 20-pack-year history of smoking appears to be the level at which significant pulmonary risk becomes apparent. A history of asthma, past episodes of respiratory failure and the presence of shortness of breath during activity are relevant in assessing a patient's pulmonary status. The characteristics and quantity of sputum production may assist the physician in distinguishing emphysema from bronchitis in patients with long-standing lung disease.

The physician should be alert for physical abnormalities that would indicate underlying respiratory disease, such as hyperinflation of the lungs, clubbing of the fingers, and discoloration of the fingers and teeth (characteristic of tobacco use). In addition, a chronic smoker will have a tobacco odor on his or her fingertips that can be detected by an astute clinician. The patient's ability to ambulate without dyspnea—although this may be confounded by his or her peripheral vascular disease—is a simple test of respiratory function. A routine chest radiograph supplements the physical examination and may screen for any acute pulmonary process.

All patients thought to be at increased risk for pulmonary complications require room air blood gas evaluation and pulmonary function tests. Oxygenation is measured by *Pao$_2$* and alveolar ventilation is assessed by *Paco$_2$*. *Forced expiratory volume* (FEV$_1$) is the volume of air exhaled in 1 second by a forced expiration after a maximal inhalation; *total volume* is the amount of air exchanged in a normal ventilatory cycle; and *functional residual capacity* (FRC) is the volume of air remaining in the lungs after a normal exhalation.

Flow rates are expressed as a volume of air expired per unit of time. These measurements are dependent on patient effort and can reveal the presence of obstructive airway disease. Flow rates are often reported as a percentage of the expected value for the patient being studied. Disease of the small airways is detected by abnormalities of the mid expiratory flow rate (FEF$_{25\%-75\%}$). This represents the midportion of the "expiration versus time" (spirogram) curve in liters per minute. FEF$_{25\%-75\%}$ is considered normal when it is greater than 80% of the predicted value or when its absolute value is 150 to 200 L/min. *Maximal voluntary ventilation,* the maximum amount of air breathed in 1 minute, generally ranges from 150 to 500 L/min and is dependent on the status of the respiratory muscles, lung compliance, and the dead space–tidal volume ratio. This test has proved to be an accurate predictor of postoperative pulmonary complications, because an abnormal value can be caused by patient debilitation as well as underlying pulmonary disease (see Table 5-1).

Patients with obstructive disease have normal vital capacity (VC) but have markedly decreased flow rates such as FEV_1 or $FEF_{25\%-75\%}$. By contrast, patients with restrictive disease have a diminished VC with *normal* expiratory flow rates. These tests are used to identify patients at high risk for postoperative pulmonary complications. For all patients with a history of chronic obstructive pulmonary disease (COPD), asthma, or chronic bronchitis, pulmonary function tests should

Table 5-1. Pulmonary Assessment

Test	Normal	High Risk
Forced expiratory volume, 1 second (FEV_1)	>80% predicted	<40%-50%
Maximal mid expiratory flow ($FEF_{25\%-75\%}$)	150-200 L/min; >80% predicted	<35%-50%
Maximal voluntary ventilation	150-500 L/min; >80% predicted	<35%-50%
Pa_{O_2}, room air	85 ± 5 mm Hg	<50-55 mm Hg
Pa_{CO_2}, room air	40 ± 4 mm Hg	>45-55 mm Hg

be performed before *and* after bronchodilator therapy to ensure optimization before surgery. Every patient should be encouraged to cease smoking for 1 to 2 weeks before surgery. Measures to optimize preoperative pulmonary function with exercises and pharmacologic manipulations have been shown to reduce the complication rate associated with COPD.

Hematologic Evaluation

An assessment of the patient's ability to form (as well as propensity for forming) thrombi must be made before *any* vascular procedure, including angiography. The history should include questions pertaining to evidence of bleeding tendencies (minor trauma, dental procedures, or previous operations), spontaneous bleeding episodes (epitaxis, easy bruising, frequent ecchymoses) and a family history of bleeding disorders. A complete list of the patient's medications is essential, because many drugs can affect platelet function (such as aspirin or anti-inflammatory agents) or coagulation capability (Coumadin). The most common laboratory tests used for screening include prothrombin time (PT), partial thromboplastin time (PTT), platelet count, and bleeding time. Any significant abnormality of these laboratory tests mandates further evaluation. This may include determination of clotting factor levels in addition to a qualified hematologic consultation.

A patient with a history of venous thrombosis or multiple graft failures should undergo a ***hypercoagulable workup*** before further vascular surgery. Although most episodes of early graft failure can be ascribed to technical errors, some patients do have a predisposition to form thrombi. Appropriate laboratory tests for this workup include measurement of protein C, protein S, anticardiolipin, antithrombin III (A-III), and lupus anticoagulant levels. Protein C is a vitamin K–dependent glycoprotein that acts at the endothelial surface to inactivate factor V_a and V_{IIIa}. Protein S is a cofactor of protein C. A level of less than 50% for protein C and less than 70% for protein S is clinically significant.

A-III binds thrombin and other activated clotting factors, especially factor X, thereby neutralizing their activity. The activity of A-III is amplified by heparin sodium. Clinical manifestations of A-III deficiency include spontaneous deep venous thrombosis and pulmonary embolism. Abnormally high heparin requirements for maintenance of a therapeutic anticoagulation level should alert the surgeon to a possible A-III deficiency. Levels of less than 60% of normal are associated with pathologic states. A-III is formed in the liver and thus hepatic insufficiency is one cause of A-III deficiency.

Lupus anticoagulant and anticardiolipin antibodies are types of antiphospholipid antibody syndromes. Lupus anticoagulant is an acquired IgG or IgM antibody that is measured by a ***Russell viper venom time.***

Anticardiolipin is also an IgG or IgM antibody measured in an *enzyme-linked immunosorbent assay* (ELISA) that contains cardiolipin as the antigen. In these patients the activated PTT is prolonged as a result of the effect of antibodies in this phospholipid-dependent assay. Clinical manifestations of these states are varied but most commonly present as recurrent venous or arterial thromboembolism. The treatment at this time for all of these hypercoagulable states is long-term anticoagulation therapy with warfarin.

Careful medical evaluation can decrease the morbidity and mortality of vascular surgery. An operation cannot be considered successful, despite its long-term patency or success in ridding the patient of his aneurysm or stenosis, if the patient's medical condition is exacerbated or he or she succumbs to cardiac or pulmonary disease.

BIBLIOGRAPHY

Blunt TJ. The role of a defined protocol for cardiac risk assessment in decreasing perioperative myocardial infarction in vascular surgery. J Vasc Surg 15:626-634, 1992.

Donaldson MC, Weinberg DS, Belkin M, Whittemore AD, Mannick JA. Screening for hypercoagulable states in vascular surgical practice: A preliminary study. J Vasc Surg 11:825-831, 1990.

Gersh BJ, Rihal CS, Rooke TW, Ballard DJ. Evaluation and management of patients with both peripheral vascular and coronary artery disease. J Am Coll Cardiol 18:203-224, 1991.

Hendel RC, Layden JJ, Leppo JA. Prognostic value of dipyridamole thallium scintigraphy for evaluation of ischemic heart disease. J Am Coll Cardiol 15:109-116, 1990.

Samlaska CP, James WD. Superficial thrombophlebitis. I. Primary hypercoagulable states. J Am Acad Dermatol 22:975-989, 1990.

6

Surgical Treatment of Lower Extremity Ischemia

Jamie Goldsmith • Clifford M. Sales • Frank J. Veith

Indications for lower extremity revascularization range from disabling claudication to limb-threatening gangrene. Although infrainguinal bypass procedures can be performed with minimal morbidity and mortality, careful consideration must be given before surgical intervention in patients with atherosclerosis that does *not* threaten a limb. Claudication, if *truly* disabling, however, remains an acceptable indication for revascularization. Patients with severe ischemia (rest pain or small patches of gangrene) in the absence of a threatened limb may be referred for evaluation. However, these patients can sometimes be managed conservatively for months or years when cardiovascular risk factors are prohibitive.

Surgical Intervention

When proceeding with revascularization, one's initial challenge is to identify the significant arterial lesion or lesions and evaluate the proximal (inflow) and distal (outflow) arterial circulation. After identification of the ischemia-producing lesions, one must determine the appropriate intervention. The basic principle for arterial bypass surgery remains the selection of an inflow site as distal as possible to provide unobstructed flow to the feet. *Percutaneous transluminal angioplasty* (PTA) of a proximal stenotic lesion is a useful adjunct procedure to increase inflow to a more distal artery. Iliac angioplasty (with or without placement of intraluminal stents) may obviate the need to use the aorta as an inflow site. The distal anastomosis is performed at a site beyond the most distal hemodynamically significant arterial lesion.

Access to the aorta may be gained by a transperitoneal or retroperitoneal approach. The retroperitoneal incision has been advocated in patients with previous abdominal surgery, obesity, or those with chronic obstructive pulmonary disease. All patients undergoing aortic procedures should have radial and pulmonary artery catheterization. A mechanical and antibiotic bowel preparation is administered preoperatively in case there is bowel ischemia or inadvertent spillage of gastrointestinal content during surgery. The use of autotransfusion limits the requirement for banked homologous blood.

Patients who are unsuitable for PTA and in whom an aortic procedure may be contraindicated because of prohibitive medical risk may undergo an extra-anatomic bypass (for example, axillofemoral or femorofemoral bypass). The axillary or contralateral femoral artery may be used as an inflow site for a bypass to a femoral artery distal to an iliac occlusion. In either instance a synthetic graft is tunneled subcutaneously through an extra-anatomic route. The artery selected for the proximal anastomosis must be carefully evaluated through angiography and noninvasive tests to diagnose unsuspected disease that may hamper inflow and cause bypass failure. The subclavian and axillary arteries are evaluated with a transfemoral or translumbar arch aortogram to diagnose unsuspected lesions. If inflow disease is present, an alternate site should be chosen for the proximal anastomosis. The site of the distal anastomosis is usually the common femoral artery, but occasionally the deep femoral or popliteal artery may be used (axillopopliteal or femoral to contralateral popliteal grafts).

Patients with lesions of the superficial femoral and/or popliteal arteries (Fig. 6-1) may be suitable candidates for a femoropopliteal bypass. The common, deep, or proximal superficial femoral arteries may be selected as the proximal inflow site. The deep femoral artery (profunda) is frequently used as the inflow site in reoperations to avoid traversing a scarred or infected groin. The popliteal artery (above- or below-knee) is used as the site for the distal anastomosis. Ideally it is important to have adequate outflow distal to the popliteal artery. However, bypasses have been successfully

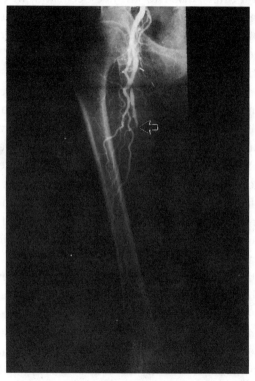

Fig. 6-1. Arteriogram showing occlusion of the femoral artery *(arrow)* with reconstitution of the popliteal artery.

performed even when the popliteal artery ends in an isolated or "blind" segment. Adequate collateral branches may arise from such blind segments to help maintain bypass patency and allow blood to flow distally.

Infrapopliteal bypass is considered a routine procedure in many centers. In the past, however, patients with a popliteal pulse and gangrenous changes in the foot were often considered candidates for primary amputation. Currently patients with infrapopliteal disease (Fig. 6-2) undergo femoral-to-distal, popliteal-to-distal (Fig. 6-3), or tibial-to-tibial bypass, as indicated. In addition to the tibial and peroneal arteries, the plantar and lateral tarsal arteries have also been used successfully as sites for distal anastomoses.

Autologous vein is the optimal graft material. Vein may be harvested from the ipsilateral greater or lesser saphenous veins. Saphenous vein may also be harvested from the contralateral leg when circulation is adequate to support healing of the surgical incision. Cephalic and basilic veins are less frequently used and may be fibrotic as a result of previous venipunctures. When autologous vein is not available or acceptable, umbilical vein and cryopreserved vein grafts have been used. At our institution, we routinely use polytetrafluoroethylene (PTFE) grafts when vein is not available. Although the use of PTFE grafts to infrapopliteal vessels remains controversial, acceptable results at several cen-

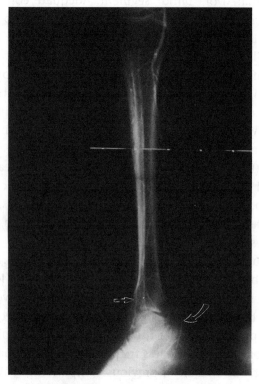

Fig. 6-2. Arteriogram showing infrapopliteal three-vessel occlusive disease with reconstitution of the posterior tibial artery *(curved arrow)* and the anterior tibial artery *(straight arrow).*

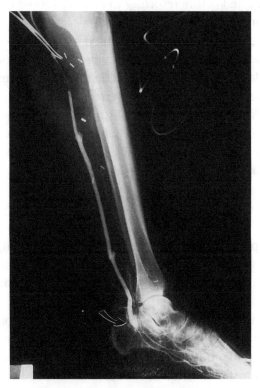

Fig. 6-3. Intraoperative arteriogram of a below-knee popliteal to posterior tibial bypass at the ankle with reversed vein graft. The bypass is shown with the distal anastomosis *(arrow)*, and flow is shown to the foot via the plantar arteries.

ters indicate that this option is feasible and should be attempted before resorting to amputation when vein is not available.

Autologous vein may be used as a graft in three ways: reversed, in situ, or nonreversed translocated (Table 6-1). In the reversed method, the vein is carefully dissected, excised, and reversed before anastomosis (so that flow is not impeded by the venous valves). The in situ method leaves the vein in place and renders the valves incompetent by the use of a valve cutter or valvulotome. The venous (side) branches are ligated to prevent formation of an arteriovenous fistula. Intra-operative angioscopy may be used to identify side branches, direct the valvulotomy, and to ensure the completeness of valve leaflet destruction. Using the nonreversed translocated method, the vein is carefully dissected and excised, and valve lysis is performed. It is similar to the in situ method, except that the vein is removed. Although each technique has its proponents, the question of which is superior has not been fully answered, and some centers are engaged in random-ized prospective studies to address this issue. To obtain optimal results, the surgeon must be proficient in all methods, since some patients are suitable candidates for only one method.

Table 6-1. Comparison of Reversed, In Situ, and Nonreversed Translocated Vein Grafts

Graft	Advantages	Disadvantages
Reversed	No valvulotome trauma Can obtain vein from another extremity Maneuverability of vein—technically easier to do anastomosis Vein can be tunneled deeply (better if wounds break down)	Vasovasorum cut Ischemia time Size mismatch*
In situ	No size mismatch Reduced ischemia time Vein well nourished	Valvulotome trauma Vein graft is more superficial Vein less mobile—technically more difficult
Nonreversed translocated saphenous vein	No size mismatch Maneuverability of vein	Vasovasorum cut Ischemia time Valvulotome trauma

*Size mismatch refers to difference in vessel diameter between vein and artery.

Acute Ischemia

Acute lower extremity ischemia is usually caused by emboli (Fig. 6-4) but may result from spontaneous thrombosis of atherosclerotic lesions. Emboli may also originate from the heart after a myocardial infarction or in patients with atrial fibrillation or in those with valvular vegetations from endocarditis. Emboli may also occur as a result of aneurysmal disease or from a diffusely atherosclerotic aorta. The presence of distal pulses and ischemic lesions of the extremities is referred to as *blue toe syndrome.* The lesions associated with these "microemboli" showered distally from a diseased aorta usually do not produce acute ischemia but, if the underlying cause (atherosclerotic aorta) is not treated, irreversible tissue necrosis can occur. In addition to emboli and thrombosis of atherosclerotic lesions, vascular trauma, bone fractures, and thrombosis of an arterial bypass graft can all produce acute limb-threatening ischemia. Acute arterial occlusion may also occur after arterial catheterization for a diagnostic or therapeutic procedure (angiography, balloon angioplasty, or placement of an intra-aortic balloon pump). Low-flow states resulting from diminished cardiac output may also lead to acutely ischemic extremities.

The timing of intervention for acute lower extremity ischemia depends on the viability of the limb at the time of examination. Prompt recognition, diagnosis,

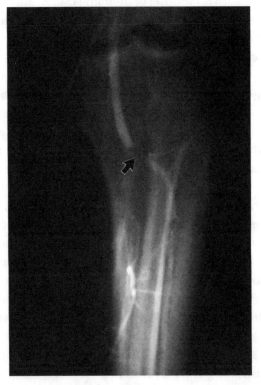

Fig. 6-4. Arteriogram showing a popliteal embolism *(arrow)* proximal to the takeoff of the anterior tibial artery.

and emergency intervention may be necessary to prevent irreversible damage and limb loss. A patient presenting with *acute* onset of disabling claudication (usually from an in situ thrombosis of a stenotic lesion) will often *not* have a threatened limb and thus immediate revascularization may not be necessary. Patients with underlying arteriosclerosis who develop acute worsening of symptoms may be less at risk for limb loss than a patient with acute limb ischemia caused by embolic disease. The preexisting collateral circulation and the more efficient oxygen extraction of the muscle place these patients at less risk for immediate limb loss. These patients can be treated with infusion of a thrombolytic agent to dissolve an intraluminal clot. Thrombolytic therapy, however, is probably contraindicated in patients with very severe, acute limb ischemia, since the time necessary for clot lysis delays restoration of blood flow and prolongs ischemia.

Loss of (or changes in) motor or sensory function in an affected limb herald the onset of *irreversible* ischemic damage. Calf tenderness indicates severe ischemia and impending muscle necrosis. This finding can be misleading and may lead to a misdiagnosis of deep vein thrombosis. Urgent arteriography is indicated, followed by operative intervention. The patient should be given intravenous heparin on admission in an effort to prevent extension of the preexisting clot. The patient should be given a bolus loading dose of 5000 U and subsequently be maintained with an activated partial thromboplastin time (PTT) of 1.5 to 2 times the control value.

Arteriography is advisable, and is especially important, in patients with preexisting arteriosclerosis. It is often difficult to distinguish between emboli and thrombi clinically or on arteriography. Angiographic characteristics of emboli include multiplicity and abrupt cutoff of the artery without the presence of collaterals. A "simple" operative Fogarty balloon catheter embolectomy may be all that is required to restore adequate blood flow. However, currently this is rarely the case with many patients who present with acute limb ischemia. Frequently these patients have advanced underlying atherosclerosis, rendering treatment difficult. Some of these patients may require an arterial bypass to save the acutely ischemic limb. The use of the p[...] teal approach to perform the embolectomy prob[...] yields better results and allows proximal access to [...] femoral and popliteal arteries as well as to the [...] distal tibial vessels. In some patients emboli are [...] and in others they are multiple (Fig. 6-5).

Once adequate flow has been restored to th[...] ed limb, a fasciotomy may be required. Fasc[...] indicated when compartment syndrome (te[...] and increased compartment pressures) occu[...] ing reperfusion of ischemic muscle. Compartme[...] sures are measured by inserting an 18-gauge [...]

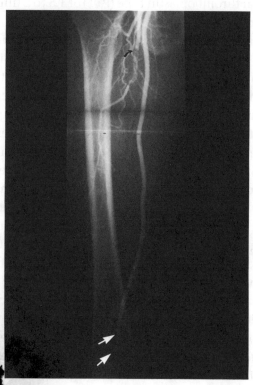

Arteriogram showing multiple emboli (profunda femoris, femoral artery) in a patient with acute ischemia. Emboli seen in deep femoral artery *(single dark arrow);* emboli superficial femoral artery *(double white arrows).*

into the anterior and posterior compartments. The catheter is attached to a pressure monitor. The normal compartment pressure is 15 to 20 mm Hg. An elevated compartment pressure over 30 mm Hg is considered an indication for fasciotomy. Elevated compartment pressure can lead to a permanent neurologic deficit in the limb and affect its viability. It should be noted that compartment syndrome can exist even in the presence of pedal pulses or can itself be a cause of acute ischemia.

Popliteal aneurysms are usually repaired electively when they reach a width of 2 cm or when they produce ischemic manifestations from thromboembolism. Thrombosis of a popliteal aneurysm (Fig. 6-6) or emboli showered distally from popliteal aneurysms may cause acute ischemia. The presence of a "bounding" or aneurysmal popliteal pulse in the contralateral limb of a patient who has acute ischemia is suggestive of this diagnosis. If the limb is not in jeopardy, infusion of a thrombolytic agent may assist in lysing the clot within the aneurysm and "open up" distally occluded vessels (Fig. 6-7). This facilitates the surgical intervention by shortening the overall length of the bypass and allowing the site of outflow to be a more proximal vessel. When the clot has been lysed in the popliteal and infrapopliteal vessels, the aneurysm may be ligated and the appropriate bypass performed.

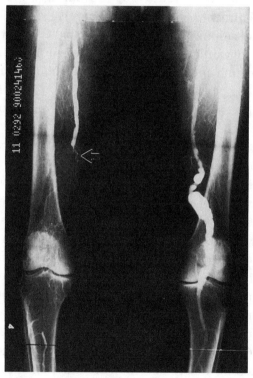

Fig. 6-6. Arteriogram showing a thrombosed popliteal aneurysm *(arrow).*

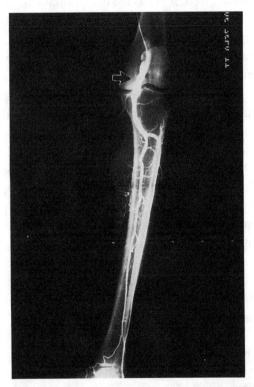

Fig. 6-7. Arteriogram showing clot lysis of a thrombosed popliteal aneurysm *(arrow)* after infusion of a thrombolytic agent.

Conclusion

Improved management of patients with limb-threatening ischemia has led to a dramatic decrease in major amputation rates. Significant advances in arteriography and surgical intervention have promoted a more aggressive approach to limb salvage surgery. Most patients (more than 98%) whose limbs are threatened because of ischemia secondary to atherosclerosis are amenable to treatment by some form of arterial bypass or balloon angioplasty. Moreover, these arterial reconstructive techniques are usually successful (more than 90%) in improving the circulation to the point at which the limb can be salvaged, although local debridement, or a toe or transmetatarsal amputation (partial or complete) may be required. Although this aggressive approach to limb salvage is complicated, often difficult, and costly, it is worthwhile for old, sick patients who generally have threatened limbs and who are not easily rehabilitated after a major lower extremity amputation.

BIBLIOGRAPHY

DeWeese JA, Leather R, Porter J. Practice guidelines: Lower extremity revascularization. J Vasc Surg 18:280-294, 1993.

Goldsmith J, Franco D, Farrell EA, Keeley J, Veith FJ. Advances in the surgical treatment of lower extremity vascular disease. J Am Acad Phys Assist 4:481-487, 1991.

Rutherford RB. Atlas of Vascular Surgery: Basic Techniques and Exposures. Philadelphia: WB Saunders, 1993.

Veith FJ. Vascular surgical techniques. In Veith FJ, Hobson RW, Williams RA, Wilson SE, eds. Vascular Surgery: Principles and Practice, 2nd ed. New York: McGraw-Hill, 1994, pp 1134-1204.

Veith FJ, Gupta SK, Samson RH, Scher LA, Fell SC, Weiss P, Janko G, Flores SW, Rifkin H, Bernstein G, Haimovici H, Gliedman ML, Sprayregen S. Progress in limb salvage by reconstructive arterial surgery combined with new or improved adjunctive procedures. Ann Surg 194:386-401, 1981.

Veith FJ, Gupta SK, Wengerter KR, Goldsmith J, Rivers SP, Bakal C, Dietzek AM, Cynamon J, Sprayregen S, Gliedman ML. Changing arteriosclerotic disease patterns and management strategies in lower-limb-threatening ischemia. Ann Surg 212:402-412, 1990.

Veith FJ, Panetta TF, Wengerter KR, Marin ML, Rivers SP, Suggs WD, Lyon RT. Femoral-popliteal-tibial occlusive disease. In Veith FJ, Hobson RW, Williams RA, Wilson SE, eds. Vascular Surgery: Principles and Practice, 2nd ed. New York: McGraw-Hill, 1994, pp 421-446.

7

Intraoperative Considerations and Adjuncts

Keith D. Calligaro

Many aspects of intraoperative monitoring and care of a patient who is undergoing a vascular operation demand attention. Since approximately 25% to 33% of patients requiring vascular surgery have significant cardiac disease, cardiovascular monitoring is obviously a critical factor to ensure a successful surgical outcome. The advantages and disadvantages of general and regional anesthesia will be discussed. One must be familiar with various drugs used in the operating room, including heparin, protamine, antibiotics, and hemostatic agents. Skin preparation and draping of the patient play important roles in preventing infection and guaranteeing adequate access to necessary inflow and outflow vessels. Mechanical retractors have recently gained widespread use, since they help to provide excellent exposure of the surgical field without requiring an assistant to struggle with hand-held retractors for long periods of time. Finally, the technique and importance of wound closure will be reviewed. All of these factors play an important role in minimizing the complication rate and increasing the chances of successfully treating these challenging patients.

Monitoring the Patient

Central monitoring devices such as central venous catheters and Swan-Ganz catheters are commonly used during vascular surgery. These instruments help to monitor the fluid and hemodynamic status of the patient. *Central venous pressure* is the systemic venous pressure measured at the level of the right atrium using a catheter advanced from a peripheral vein into the superior vena cava or right atrium. However, central venous pressure reflects only right atrial filling pressure and right ventricular performance. The *pulmonary arterial diastolic* or *pulmonary capillary wedge pressure* is a better estimate of left heart function and fluid status than is central venous pressure. A flow directed catheter is introduced from a peripheral vein (usually the internal jugular or subclavian) and advanced through the right side of the heart into the pulmonary artery. Swan-Ganz catheters can provide measurement of cardiac output, mixed venous (pulmonary arterial) oxygen saturation, and volume status of the patient. Swan-Ganz catheters are frequently used for aortic procedures and lower extremity bypasses in patients with significant cardiac risk factors. Cardiac optimization with the use of a Swan-Ganz catheter generally requires 12 to 24 hours of preoperative monitoring. These catheters are rarely necessary for carotid artery operations, since these procedures can usually be completed in 2 to 3 hours, fluid shifts are minimal, and most patients will tolerate a regular diet the day after surgery.

Arterial lines are placed in many patients who are undergoing vascular surgery to monitor blood pressure continuously and to obtain arterial blood gas levels and perform other necessary blood tests. An arterial line is essential during carotid and aortic operations to detect any precipitous changes in blood pressure. Many vascular patients not only have significant obstructive disease in their coronary and lower extremity arteries but also in their upper extremities. Careful attention should be given to ensure patency of both the radial and ulnar arteries before cannulation of either artery by using the Allen test. Use of a brachial arterial line should be avoided whenever possible, since collateralization around the brachial artery may be inadequate to prevent hand ischemia if the catheter causes arterial thrombosis.

Continuous intraoperative monitoring of the electrocardiogram is essential to detect dysrhythmias or significant bradycardia or tachycardia. It is important to discuss placement of the cardiac leads with the anesthesiologist so they are not included in the operative field, especially before surgery of the thoracic aorta or subclavian and axillary arteries. A pulse oximeter is placed on a finger to measure arterial oxygen saturation noninvasively.

A Foley catheter is routinely inserted for all vascular operations to monitor urine output and assess intravascular volume. A nasogastric tube is used for all abdominal aortic or retroperitoneal operations to prevent gastric distention and pulmonary aspiration and to reduce postoperative ileus.

Skin Preparation and Draping of the Patient

Although studies in the literature have shown conflicting results, most have demonstrated the superiority of a betadine skin preparation over an alcohol-based preparation to decrease the potential for infection. The only instance in which we use an alcohol-based preparation is when the patient has a known allergy to iodine. The skin should be shaved with a clipper or a razor in a preparation room immediately before the operation or in the operating room after the patient is anesthetized.

It is critical that any area of the body in which access to an inflow or outflow artery may be required be included in the prepared field. For a carotid endarterectomy, areas that must be prepared include the midline of the neck, the clavicle, the lower border of

the mandible, and the lower part of the earlobe to
ensure adequate proximal and distal exposure of the
common and internal carotid arteries and to provide
useful anatomic landmarks. Towels are placed along
the midline of the neck, below the clavicle, across the
lower face, and along the lateral neck so the previously
mentioned landmarks are within the operative field.
The towels can be secured to the skin with staples or
with adhesive plastic drapes. The remainder of the
body is draped with sterile sheets. A folded sterile sheet
is placed across the rest of the head and arms and
secured to IV poles to provide a sterile barrier between
the surgical field and the anesthesiologist.

For an axillofemoral bypass, sites to be prepared
include the clavicle, the chest below the clavicle, the
ipsilateral upper extremity, flank, groin, and upper
thigh. Towels can be stapled to the skin to mark these
borders, and sterile drapes are then placed to cover the
rest of the body.

The patient should be supine for all vascular operations, except when repair of a thoracoabdominal aneurysm or a retroperitoneal approach is planned. In
the former case, the patient should be placed in the
right lateral decubitus position with the aid of an
inflatable cushion. The hips should be as flat as possible to ensure easy access to the femoral arteries. A
shoulder roll is placed under the right axilla to prevent
brachial nerve palsy. Access to the aorta by a left retro-

peritoneal approach is aided by placing a small towel roll under the left flank. The patient is placed in a reverse jackknife position to allow for extension of the flank and provide better exposure of the retroperitoneum and aorta.

For an abdominal or lower extremity procedure, a folded towel is placed over the pubis and the edges of a towel stapled to the surrounding skin to isolate this area from the operative field. For abdominal aortic operations, the skin between the lower half of the chest and the midthighs should be prepared. If an aortic bypass for occlusive disease is planned, it is prudent to include both lower extremities in the operative field in case a bypass or thromboembolectomy of a leg proves necessary.

For a lower extremity bypass, areas to be prepared include the lower half of the abdomen, the contralateral groin, and the entire ipsilateral leg. This extensive skin preparation allows for use of the proximal external iliac artery, contralateral femoral artery, or distal arteries of the leg as inflow or outflow vessels. If there is any question about the adequacy of the ipsilateral greater saphenous vein for use as a conduit for an arterial bypass, the contralateral leg and one arm should be prepared to ensure that an acceptable length of vein can be procured. Preoperative duplex mapping of the superficial veins usually provides reliable information concerning vein adequacy and avoids the need for uniformly preparing both legs and one arm. At least one assistant is required to raise the leg by holding the foot during skin preparation for a lower extremity bypass so that the posterior aspect of the leg can be prepared.

Mechanical Assistants

The use of mechanical retractors or "robot retractors" has greatly aided in providing continuous exposure of the operative field. It is critical that constant and stable exposure of an artery be provided while it is dissected and during construction of an anastomosis. Retraction of adjacent soft tissues is usually best provided by these mechanical retractors. These devices are less tiring and more reliable than an intern to retract adjacent tissue. An Omni retractor provides excellent exposure for abdominal aortic operations. The small bowel is packed toward the right abdominal gutter and the transverse colon and omentum are packed cephalad into the left upper quadrant.

A single-armed robot retractor can be used to gain excellent exposure of the cephalad portion of the internal carotid, the distal external iliac or the proximal common femoral arteries. The robot-retractor is usually placed on the side opposite the operative field so that the vertical pole is not in the way of the operating surgeon.

Type of Anesthesia

Although a general anesthetic is universally given for abdominal aortic operations, controversy exists about the benefit of general anesthesia rather than epidural or spinal anesthesia for lower extremity bypasses. Although one might assume that a regional anesthetic causes less cardiac stress than a general anesthetic, several studies have documented that this is not necessarily true. Spinal and epidural anesthesia cause peripheral vasodilation, which often requires fluid loading to maintain blood pressure. This additional fluid may lead to increased left ventricular workload and pulmonary edema. Therefore there *may* be potential advantages to the use of a regional anesthetic compared with a general anesthetic for a patient with poor pulmonary function or for a patient undergoing a carotid endarterectomy, where neurologic function can be assessed because the patient is conscious.

Drugs Used in the Operating Room

Heparin is routinely used during vascular operations, with the possible exception of repair of a thoracoabdominal aneurysm. We prefer to follow the anticoagulant effect of heparin closely by frequent monitoring of the activated clotting time (ACT). Although a PTT more accurately reflects the anticoagulation effect of this drug, most laboratories require an hour to run this test. The advantage of an ACT test is that it can be performed in the operating room in less than 10 minutes. Although most pharmacology textbooks state than an ACT reflects an anticoagulated state when it is greater than 150 seconds, we prefer a level between 200 and 250 seconds. We administer heparin as a 100 mg/kg bolus if the baseline ACT is less than 150 seconds. As a general rule we give 1000 U of heparin as a bolus every hour but modify the dose based on the ACT.

If unexplained arterial or graft thrombosis occurs intraoperatively or in the immediate postoperative period, in the absence of technical errors, a rapid investigation of certain hypercoagulable states should be performed. An appropriately elevated ACT after heparin administration effectively rules out antithrombin III deficiency. Heparin acts by activating antithrombin III, and this protein then inhibits certain clotting factors, causing a subsequent rise in the ACT. If the ACT remains normal after an appropriate heparin bolus, antithrombin III deficiency must be considered.

A known side effect of heparin is that the drug paradoxically can cause clotting. If a patient has antibodies that become activated by heparin, the antibodies may cause platelet aggregation with subsequent arterial thrombosis. This hypercoagulable state is called *heparin-induced thrombocytopenia.* If unexplained clotting occurs, a platelet count should be obtained immediately to rule out this condition.

Protamine can be administered to reverse the anti-coagulant effect of heparin. The recommended dose is 1 mg protamine/100 U of heparin if the heparin bolus was given in the past 30 minutes and 0.5 mg/100 U of heparin if heparin was given more than 30 minutes previously. Side effects of protamine include hypotension, bradycardia, and even cardiac arrest. These reactions may be particularly likely to occur in diabetics taking NPH insulin, since they may develop an allergic reaction to protamine (the *P* in NPH stands for protamine).

The efficacy of prophylactic antibiotics has been well documented in several prospective, randomized trials in decreasing wound infections in patients undergoing vascular surgery. A first-generation cephalosporin such as cefazolin is currently the antibiotic of choice. The most important dose is the preoperative one, which consists of 1 g administered intravenously about 30 minutes before the skin incision. The antibiotic should be given every 4 hours intraoperatively for lengthy operations and continued every 8 hours postoperatively for up to 48 hours. Many authorities recommend only the preoperative and intraoperative doses and believe postoperative doses are unnecessary. If the patient is receiving other antibiotics for a concomitant foot infection, and if these antibiotics provide broad-spectrum coverage of most gram positive and gram negative bacteria, then cefazolin is not required. Prospective, randomized studies have documented the benefit of local wound irrigation before closure of the wound when intravenous antibiotics were not given. Although local wound irrigation provided no statistically significant benefit if intravenous antibiotics were also administered, we currently recommend copious irrigation of all wounds before they are closed, since infection of a graft is a devastating complication.

Hemostatic agents such as thrombin, Gelfoam, Avitene, and Surgicel can speed hemostasis of an anastomosis once the clamps are released and blood flow is restored through a graft. We prefer Surgicel because of its equal efficacy, ease of handling, and lower cost compared with other hemostatic agents.

Wound Closure

Meticulous wound closure is essential to ensure that the wound will heal and to prevent wound dehiscence and infection. When closing a neck incision after a carotid endarterectomy, we prefer to reapproximate the sternocleidomastoid muscle with a few interrupted sutures and close the platysma with a running absorbable suture. Although closing the skin with staples is faster, we recommend using a running subcuticular absorbable suture for cosmetic reasons. Leg incisions should be closed in multiple layers, including the fascia, subcutaneous, and skin layers. Particular attention should be paid during closure of groin incisions, since this site is most commonly associated with wound and graft infections. The use of skip incisions for greater saphenous vein harvesting greatly facilitates appropriate skin closure. Careful closure should be performed on the crural fascia, Scarpa's fascia, subcutaneous tissue, and skin. Before the drapes are removed, the wounds should be covered with sterile dressings.

BIBLIOGRAPHY

Bunt TJ. Synthetic vascular graft infections. I. Graft infections. Surgery 6:733-746, 1983.

Pearce WH. Perioperative monitoring and intensive care of patients undergoing major vascular surgery. In Rutherford RB, ed. Vascular Surgery, 3rd ed. Philadelphia: WB Saunders, 1989, pp 364-374.

Robertson JM, Buckberg GD. Cardiovascular monitoring and perioperative management of the vascular surgery patient. In Moore W, ed. Vascular Surgery: A Comprehensive Review. New York: Grune & Stratton, 1986, pp 317-337.

8

Postoperative Care After Lower Extremity Revascularization

Elizabeth A. Farrell

Postoperative Monitoring

Although the focus of the surgeon's attention in the postoperative period will be on the revascularized extremity, it is imperative that careful attention be paid to the cardiopulmonary system as well. Patients with peripheral vascular disease frequently have other manifestations of atherosclerosis including concomitant coronary artery disease. This extravascular involvement places these patients at greatly increased risk for myocardial ischemia and subsequent infarction. Thus cardiac enzyme (creatine phosphokinase [CPK-MB], serum glutamate oxaloacetate transaminase [SGOT], and lactic dehydrogenase [LDH]) and electrocardiographic evaluation must be performed routinely (every 8 hours for 24 hours) after all lower extremity revascularizations. Judicious fluid administration is important in the immediate postoperative period, with careful consideration of the cardiac and renal function of the patient. Atherosclerotic involvement of the kidneys or diabetic nephropathy is common in the vascular surgery patient, rendering achievement of appropriate fluid balance even more difficult. Additional difficulties may be encountered with aortic procedures, because fluid shifts can be massive following these operations. Extravasation of fluid into the extravascular space during the course of the operation is followed by resorption of fluid back into the intravascular compartment approximately 48 hours postoperatively. A patient with compromised cardiac function may be unable to tolerate this large fluid infusion and severe congestive heart failure may ensue. Therefore close monitoring must extend at least 72 hours postoperatively, including monitoring of central pressures, urine output, and serum electrolytes; careful physical examination should also be performed, particularly regarding the lungs.

Once the patient is extubated, aggressive pulmonary toilet must be encouraged to prevent atelectasis and pneumonia. A deterioration in the patient's mental status may be the initial sign of compromised respiratory function (hypoxia). A careful investigation must be implemented to establish the cause of an altered mental status, including arterial blood gas determinations, electrocardiogram, cardiac enzyme measurements, assessment of medications and, if necessary, a CT scan of the brain. Although most vascular surgery patients are elderly and highly susceptible to "ICU psychosis" (confusion associated with the loss of day and night differentiation as a result of constant monitoring and sleep deprivation), it is dangerous to initially ascribe an altered mental status to this more "benign" condition. Rather, the diagnosis of ICU psychosis should be one of exclusion after the more immediately threatening diagnoses such as infection, electrolyte imbalance, hypoxia, hypotension and ischemia are ruled out.

Anticoagulation and Antiplatelet Agents

The use of anticoagulants and antiplatelet agents is relatively common in vascular surgery. The indications vary widely; however, the basic principle is to prolong graft patency. Antiplatelet agents (aspirin, dipyridamole [Persantine], or ticlopidine HCl) are routinely administered to all patients undergoing arterial reconstruction during the preoperative and postoperative periods. Low-molecular-weight dextran has been shown to be effective in the immediate postoperative period and can be administered intravenously for the first 2 postoperative days. Long-term anticoagulation with heparin followed by warfarin sodium should be instituted in all patients with embolic disease as well as those with infrapopliteal synthetic grafts.

Heparin is administered intravenously and has a half-life of 1.5 hours. Therapeutic values are determined by monitoring either the activated clotting time (ACT) or the partial thromboplastin time (PTT), both of which should be in the range of 1.5 to 2.0 times the normal or baseline value. Heparin inhibits clotting by a number of mechanisms. The conversion of prothrombin to thrombin is inhibited, thereby preventing the degradation of fibrinogen to fibrin (thrombin is a necessary factor for this reaction to occur). Heparin also *enhances* the activity of antithrombin III—a compound that inhibits the activity of thrombin and thus impedes the degradation of fibrinogen into fibrin. Heparin can also inhibit platelet aggregation, thereby preventing the formation of platelet plugs.

The effects of heparin are reversed by intravenous administration of protamine sulfate, although great care must be taken, because severe hypotensive reactions are not uncommon when this drug is administered, particularly in insulin-dependent diabetics.

Coumadin is an oral anticoagulant with a half-life of 36 to 72 hours. Therapeutic levels are thought to be attained when the prothrombin time (PT) ranges from 1.5 to 2 times the control value. Its anticoagulant effects are achieved by interfering with the synthesis of the vitamin K–dependent factors II, VII, IX, and X. After cessation of coumadin administration, 4 to 5 days may be required before the anticoagulation effect is abolished. Vitamin K (either intravenous or intramuscular) or fresh frozen plasma may be administered for a more rapid normalization of the anticoagulant effects.

Aspirin, at a low dose, prevents platelet aggregation, and its effects last approximately 7 days. The mechanism of action is through suppression of the enzyme, cyclo-oxygenase, which is necessary for the production of both thromboxane A_2 (TXA_2) and prostaglandin I_2 (PGI_2). TXA_2 is synthesized by the platelet and is a potent stimulator of platelet aggregation. The synthesis of PGI_2, a potent antagonist of platelet aggregation produced by the ***endothelial cell,*** is also suppressed as a result of cyclo-oxygenase inhibition. The endothelial cell, however, has the ability to recover from the effects of aspirin, whereas the effects on platelets remain for the life of that cell.

Dipyridamole (Persantine) interferes with platelet aggregation by inhibiting the action of cAMP phosphodiesterase—an enzyme which inactivates platelet cyclic adenosine phosphate (cAMP). This monophosphate increase in cAMP acts to inhibit platelet aggregation, and this antithrombotic effect may be synergistic with aspirin.

Dextran is a long-chain carbohydrate that is available in varying molecular weights. Dextran 40 and dextran 70 (molecular weight 40,000 or 70,000 daltons) are the commonly used preparations. Although the exact nature of the antithrombotic properties is incompletely understood, dextran appears to reduce platelet adhesiveness and aggregation. It also decreases blood viscosity and potentiates the lysis of thrombi.

Intravenous infusion of low molecular weight dextran (dextran 40) should begin in the immediate postoperative period. No more than 1 L/day should be administered, and the infusion should be discontinued before the second postoperative day. Adverse reactions, including renal failure or anaphylaxis, are rare and usually occur at the start of infusion. Fluid overload may occur as a result of the plasma-expanding properties of dextran. Therefore close monitoring of fluid status and cardiac function is mandatory in patients receiving this solution.

Graft Evaluation

Postoperative assessment of the revascularized limb includes evaluation for patency as well as postoperative complications such as hematoma, infection, or venous thrombosis. The presence of distal pulses and the location of a palpable graft pulse should be noted in the operating room and carefully followed in the postoperative period. It is not uncommon for the revascularized limb to develop edema that will persist for several months after surgery. A limb that was cool and cyanotic preoperatively should be warmer and demonstrate a pinker hue after successful revascularization.

The presence of a pulse distal to a bypass graft signifies a patent graft. The ability to palpate a distal pulse depends on the skill of the examiner, the anatomic location of the distal anastomosis, and the distal arterial runoff. Although a bypass to an anterior tibial artery with straight line flow to the foot usually produces a palpable dorsalis pedal pulse, a bypass to the peroneal artery, not anatomically situated to enable palpation, may not yield a palpable distal pulse. However, with good runoff via collaterals, the patient may regain a dorsalis pedis pulse.

The initial postoperative examination should specify the exact procedure, including the anatomic positioning of the graft, the proximal and distal anastomoses, the type of graft material, complications, findings of the intraoperative angiogram, and the pulse status. It is not uncommon for distal pulses to be absent initially, only to become palpable several hours later. This is a result of arterial spasm from the intraoperative manipulation of the vessels. If, however, a distal pulse was initially noted and can no longer be palpated, further investigation is necessary. Noninvasive procedures can be used to evaluate the status of the bypass graft. These include pulse volume recordings (PVRs), segmental Doppler–determined ankle pressures, and duplex ultrasound examinations. PVRs should be obtained preoperatively (baseline) and immediately postoperatively (postoperative baseline) and should be repeated thereafter if there is a question about graft patency.

Duplex ultrasound examination of a bypass graft should be obtained within 1 week of the initial bypass procedure and repeated periodically. The duplex scan measures flow velocity and can visualize flow disturbances, stenotic lesions, retained valves, pseudoaneurysms, and arteriovenous fistulas within the by-pass graft. These tests are routinely performed every 4 to 6 months; however, development of ischemic symptoms or a change in the pulse examination warrants more urgent examination.

An abnormal duplex scan or a reappearance of ischemic symptoms necessitates the performance of an arteriogram. Although the arteriogram remains the gold standard for assessing the status of a bypass graft, its invasive nature limits its use only to those situations that by clinical or duplex criteria would necessitate intervention. A *failing* bypass graft is one that has not yet thrombosed but is threatened, and if left untreated, will close. The identification of a graft in this state necessitates an arteriogram to define the nature of the failing graft lesion. The arteriogram may reveal a focal graft stenosis or a widely patent bypass graft throughout. However, progression of disease in the inflow or outflow vessels may be the cause of the deterioration of graft function. In any event, the threatening lesion that is causing decreased flow through the bypass should be corrected.

Early Graft Failure

Thrombosis of a bypass graft within 30 days of its placement is termed *early graft failure.* It is presumed that early graft failure is caused by problems with the graft itself, the anastomoses, or the inflow or outflow

vessels. An arteriogram is usually obtained in the operating room after thrombectomy to establish the reason
for the graft thrombosis. Frequently observed causes
of early graft failure include retained valves in an in
situ bypass graft or inadequate outflow. If a graft originates distal to an unappreciated stenosis, the increased
flow resulting from the bypass graft can make a previously insignificant stenosis hemodynamically compromising, thereby limiting graft inflow and contributing to early thrombosis. A poorly tunneled graft or
one whose length is excessive can result in twisting
or kinking of the graft. A technically suboptimal anastomosis can also cause early graft failure.

The approach to managing the failed bypass graft
is dependent upon the cause of failure and the conduit
material. Autologous saphenous vein maintains its
viability from nutrients within the circulating blood.
Therefore *prompt* repair is necessary to ensure secondary patency. Synthetic grafts can withstand longer
intervals of occlusion without impacting negatively
on secondary patency.

An alternative method to the established technique of operative thrombectomy is the use of thrombolytic therapy—specifically, urokinase. Although
thrombolytic therapy may be useful in restoring graft
patency, it will not correct the underlying pathologic
factors responsible for graft failure. The utility of this
therapeutic modality lies in its ability to remove the
thrombus from within the graft, thereby accurately

demonstrating the cause for graft thrombosis. A major limitation to the use of urokinase in these circumstances is the significant risk of hemorrhage from newly formed suture lines and raw surgical surfaces. Therefore it is important to carefully assess the specific situation when deciding upon a method for treating early graft failure.

Infections

Despite meticulous adherence to sterile technique, wound infections do occur. The diagnosis is made on physical examination when the wound is erythematous, indurated, and warm and the patient develops a fever. Fluctuance, skin-edge breakdown, and purulent drainage are other signs of wound infection. Early recognition of wound infections and institution of appropriate therapy (aggressive drainage, local wound care, and intravenous antibiotics) can help to prevent the wound infection from involving the bypass graft.

Graft infections may result from extension of an adjacent wound infection, although direct bacterial seeding of the graft (at the time of operation or subsequently) represents another mechanism. The delivery of adequate levels of antibiotics and aggressive debridement and wound care are essential to the management of infected wounds. Although prosthetic graft preservation is controversial, excellent results have been obtained with graft-preserving forms of treatment provided that the patient does not have septicemia, the anastomoses are intact, and the graft is patent. This may result in a large, open defect with an exposed bypass graft in the base of the wound. Special care must be taken to debride all necrotic tissue and to provide moist antibiotic dressings over the exposed graft in an effort to allow for the overgrowth of healthy granulation tissue. A rotational muscle flap can be employed to hasten the covering of an exposed bypass graft. If the graft is thrombosed, it should be excised leaving only a small stump on the native artery, thereby avoiding the need to occlude a patent artery that is maintaining limb viability. If the graft must be removed and the native artery must be interrupted, an extra-anatomic bypass is often necessary to restore adequate blood supply while avoiding the currently infected wound. Such restoration of a blood supply will allow for viability of the tissue distal to the graft as well as aid in wound healing.

Additional Postoperative Considerations

Wound healing following lower extremity revascularization demands special attention. The skin closure must be performed with attention to detail as incisional breakdown is more likely given the relatively ischemic nature of the limb. Postoperative swelling of the revascularized limb can exert tension on the suture line, further compromising the healing process. Incisions performed in previously operated regions are at an even greater risk of breakdown and infection.

Care of gangrenous lesions or amputation sites can add to the complexity of postoperative management. Open wounds should be dressed with wet-to-dry dressings using normal saline. Removing the dressing after it has dried (*not* rewetting it prior to removal) will aid in the mechanical debridement of a wound. The use of a wet-to-wet dressing (continuous moistening of a dressing) will prevent desiccation, promote drainage, and help to heal precarious wounds in ischemic limbs. Such dressings must be applied carefully, ensuring that only the wound be covered by the wet gauze to avoid maceration of the surrounding tissue. Placement of adhesive tape directly on the skin should be avoided, since it can cause skin breakdown.

Frequent bedside debridements of necrotic tissue should be performed. Many patients are able to tolerate this seemingly painful procedure, because their diabetic neuropathy has produced an insensate foot. Hydrotherapy (whirlpool treatments) can mechanically debride wounds and this should be performed on a regular basis. Successful wound management necessitates frequent debridements of necrotic tissue to control infection and obtain healing.

Although nutritional status is given a great deal of attention in general surgical patients, assessment of this is often overlooked in patients undergoing a vascular surgical procedure. Measurement of serum albumin and total lymphocyte count and anergy testing are simple tests of nutritional status. Malnutrition can occur in vascular patients because of the chronic nature of their disease, depression, or loss of appetite caused by severe rest pain.

Rehabilitation of the vascular surgery patient is an integral part of patient care. Most patients are elderly and become rapidly deconditioned during even short periods of bed confinement. This is exacerbated by the incisional pain that accompanies the long incisions of distal revascularization procedures. Institution of physical therapy early in the postoperative period hastens the return of these patients to a functional state. It is also necessary for amputees to be properly fitted with prosthetic devices or custom shoes to aid in proper balancing during ambulation.

Care of the vascular surgery patient in the postoperative period mandates attention to detail. The surgeon must orchestrate the care of the patient and involve many different specialists. Attention must be directed not only toward the graft and the incisions but toward the patient's overall condition—both physical and emotional. Astute postoperative care clearly improves long-term results of distal arterial reconstructive surgery.

BIBLIOGRAPHY

Boucher CA, Brewster DC, Darling RC, Okada RD, Strauss HW, Polost GM. Determination of cardiac risk by dipyridamole-thallium imaging before peripheral vascular surgery. N Engl J Med 312:389-394, 1985.

Calligaro KD, Veith FJ, Schwartz ML, Savarese RP, Goldsmith J, Westcott CJ, DeLaurentis DA. When is it safe to leave an infected prosthetic arterial graft in place? In Veith FJ, ed. Current Critical Problems in Vascular Surgery, vol 4. St. Louis: Quality Medical Publishing, 1992, pp 365-370

DePalma RG. Patterns of Peripheral Atherosclerosis: Developments, Complications and Treatment. Amsterdam: Elsevier Science, 1987, pp 161-172.

Flinn WR, Rohrer MJ, Yao JST, McCarthy WJ, Fahey VA, Bergan JJ. Improved long-term patency of infragenicular polytetrafluoroethylene grafts. J Vasc Surg 7:685-690, 1988.

Goldsmith J, Franco CD, Farrell EA, Keeley J, Veith FJ. Advances in the surgical treatment of lower extremity vascular disease. J Am Acad Phys Assist 4:481-487, 1991.

Rutherford RB, Jones DN, Bergentz SE, Bergquist D, Karmody AM, Dardik H, Moore WS, Goldstone J, Flinn WR, Comeroth AJ, Fry WJ, Shah PM. The efficacy of dextran 40 in preventing early postoperative thrombosis following difficult lower extremity bypass. J Vasc Surg 25:765-773, 1984.

Veith FJ, Gupta SK, Ascer E, Flores, SW, Samson RH, Scher LA, Towne JB, Bernhard VM, Bonier P, Flinn WR, Astleford P, Yao JST, Bergan JJ. Six-year prospective multicenter randomized comparison of autologous saphenous vein graft and expanded polytetrafluoroethylene grafts in infrainguinal arterial reconstructions. J Vasc Surg 3:104-114, 1986.

Veith FJ, Gupta SK, Samson RH, Scher LA, Fell SC, Weiser P, Janko G, Flores SW, Rifkin H, Bernstein G, Haimovici H, Gleidman ML. Progress in limb salvage by reconstructive arterial surgery combined with new or improved adjunctive procedures. Ann Surg 194:386-401, 1981.

Veith FJ, Weiser RK, Gupta SK, Scher LA, Samson RH, Ascer E, White-Flores S, Sprayregen S. Diagnosis and management of failing lower extremity arterial reconstructions prior to graft occlusion. J Cardiovasc Surg 25:381-384, 1984.

9

Diseases of the Aorta and the Visceral Arteries

Luis A. Sanchez

Aneurysmal Disease

ABDOMINAL AORTA. An aneurysm is best defined as a *permanent increase in arterial diameter* of greater than 50% of the normal artery. Abdominal aortic aneurysms (AAAs) most commonly arise below the level of the renal arteries. Seventy percent of AAAs involve the iliac arteries and only 2% extend proximally to involve the renal or visceral vessels. The recognized incidence of infrarenal AAAs (1.8% to 6.6%) has more than doubled over the last 20 years, owing mostly (but not entirely) to improvement in diagnostic imaging techniques. The incidence of *symptomatic* abdominal aortic aneurysms has also more than doubled over the same period and the mortality associated with these lesions has increased. Despite this real increase in incidence, AAA remains predominantly a disease affecting men (3.8:1), and the condition continues to show a strong family predisposition.

Etiologic factors. The cause of most AAAs was previously thought to be atherosclerosis. AAA pathogenesis is now believed to be related to a complex set of genetic, environmental, and biochemical factors that act in concert to alter connective tissue metabolism. There is a frequent association of AAAs with other peripheral aneurysms. The genetic influence of the disease is evident in the familial distribution often seen with AAAs. Several biochemical studies have suggested increased elastase activity and a decreased alpha-1-antitrypsin level (a major elastase inhibitor) in these patients. Abnormal collagen metabolism has also been implicated as a possible etiologic factor, although atherosclerosis remains the most common cause of AAA. Other less common etiologic factors include trauma, infection (syphilis and salmonella arteritis), and connective tissue disorders (Ehlers-Danlos and Marfan's syndrome).

Diagnosis. Most aortoiliac aneurysms are asymptomatic (75%) and are found when the patient is examined for an unrelated condition. AAAs are asymptomatic unless acute expansion or disruption of the wall occurs. Patients with a symptomatic AAA may present with syncope, pain (abdominal, flank, or back), and hypotension. Less often, they present with signs of partial intestinal obstruction as the duodenum is stretched over the enlarging aneurysm. Mucosal hemorrhage from the duodenal wall will produce gastrointestinal bleeding. Erosion of the opposing walls of the duodenum and aorta will produce massive bleeding from an aortoduodenal fistula. An aortocaval fistula (erosion of the AAA into the inferior vena cava) produces an abdominal bruit, venous hypertension, edema, and heart failure. This unusual entity may result in renal failure (secondary to ureteral obstruction), distal embolization of aortic debris, or aortic thrombosis.

A carefully performed physical examination can be valuable in the diagnosis of AAAs. It is accurate in more than 80% of cases if the patient's abdominal girth is less than 100 cm. When palpable, the aneurysm is felt *at or above* the level of the umbilicus as this is the point of the abdominal aorta bifurcation. However, the physical examination can be misleading. A nonaneurysmal ectatic aorta or a normal aorta in a thin lordotic patient can be palpated and mistaken for an AAA. Pulsations from a normal aorta may be transmitted through another intra-abdominal mass that lies anterior or lateral to the aorta. Most important is that an AAA may not be palpable in an obese patient or one with a distended abdomen. When assessing a palpable aorta, both lateral extents of the vessel must be palpable. Many patients will have intact distal pulses in the presence of an abdominal aneurysm. It is imperative that these pulses be carefully assessed at the time of presentation, since aneurysmal disease (aortic or peripheral) may present with distal embolization.

Radiographic evaluation is imperative in the assessment of patients with suspected AAAs. Plain abdominal films may demonstrate the calcified aneurysmal wall. The most commonly used screening modality for the abdominal aortic aneurysm is an abdominal ultrasound examination. The test is accurate, simple to perform, and relatively inexpensive. Unfortunately, the effectiveness of the test is limited by the presence of bowel gas and its inability to provide information consistently about the proximal and distal extent of the aneurysm.

Computed tomography (CT) is highly accurate for visualizing the aneurysmal abdominal aorta (Fig. 9-1). Abdominal CT scanning is superior to ultrasonography in its ability to identify extravasation of blood when a diagnosis of ruptured aneurysm is suspected. It will also identify venous anomalies, renal anomalies, the

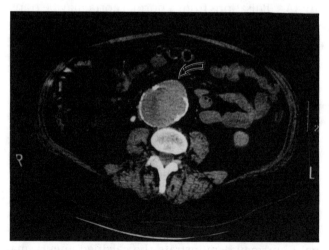

Fig. 9-1. Abdominal CT showing a 6.3 cm calcified infrarenal abdominal aortic aneurysm (AAA) with an anterior bulge *(arrow)* at the noncalcified portion of the aneurysm.

extent of the aneurysm, the degree and location of calcific aortic plaques, and the presence of other intra-abdominal pathologic conditions. Additionally, it is the best preoperative study for identifying retroperitoneal fibrosis and inflammatory AAAs.

Angiography, conventional or digital, is no longer "required" before repair of an AAA. Although many surgeons continue to use angiography routinely, citing the added information gained in as many as one third of cases, its inherent risks must be appreciated (Fig. 9-2). Specific indications have been suggested for the selective use of preoperative aortography:

- Associated renovascular hypertension (suspected or documented)
- Unexplained impaired renal function
- Suspected aneurysmal extension to juxtarenal or suprarenal levels
- Symptoms of visceral angina
- Unexplained flank or abdominal bruit
- Diminished femoral pulses
- Symptoms of peripheral vascular occlusive disease
- Horseshoe kidney
- Chronic aortic dissection
- Iliac artery aneurysms

Magnetic resonance arteriography and spiral CT scanning are new noninvasive diagnostic modalities that create anatomic images in multiple planes. The role of these new technologies is promising but remains to be evaluated.

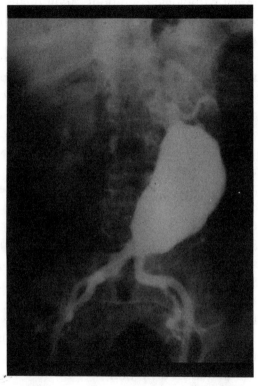

Fig. 9-2. Aortogram showing a large infrarenal AAA extending to the aortic bifurcation and bowing to the left of the spine as the aorta enlarged and elongated.

Treatment indications. The repair of AAAs is indicated when they thrombose, embolize to the distal circulation, cause symptoms by local effects on the surrounding structures, or are associated with a fistula to the venous system or enteral conduits. These indications appear infrequently, since the majority (75%) of AAAs are asymptomatic at the time of presentation. Indications for operative intervention in an asymptomatic patient relate to the prevention of rupture, with its associated high mortality. The risk of aneurysmal rupture is related to the size of the aneurysm, its rate of growth, and the presence of symptoms. The 5-year risk of rupture for a 4 cm aneurysm is less than 15%, while for an 8 cm aneurysm the risk is greater than 75%. It is generally agreed that at 5 to 6 cm, the risk of AAA rupture is substantially increased so that it exceeds the surgical risk for most patients. Factors increasing the risk of aneurysm rupture include a rapid growth rate (greater than 0.4 cm/year), hypertension, generalized arterial ectasia, and chronic obstructive pulmonary disease.

Although the magnitude of the operation for repair of an AAA must be appreciated, the patient's chance for survival when the repair is attempted for a *ruptured* AAA is significantly less. The chance of survival after the repair of a ruptured AAA averages 45%, and for patients presenting in shock with free intra-abdominal rupture, it is less than 10%. The mortality associated with an elective aneurysm repair is 3% to 5% and is usually related to the patient's coexisting medical conditions. Age *alone* is not an exclusion criterion. When AAA size exceeds 5 cm, most surgeons would concur that repair of the aneurysm is indicated in all but the highest risk patients, because the risk of rupture and the associated mortality exceed the surgical risk.

Controversy exists about preoperative evaluation for elective AAA repair. Some have suggested that an asymptomatic patient with a normal physical examination and ECG can safely undergo AAA repair without further cardiac workup. Others include the use of noninvasive studies for all patients because of the high prevalence of coronary artery disease (CAD) in patients with aneurysmal disease (20%). All agree that patients with symptomatic cardiac disease should undergo preoperative noninvasive cardiac evaluation (dipyridamole-thallium scan, echocardiography, or ejection fraction evaluation). Patients whose studies confirm the presence of CAD should undergo cardiac catheterization and correction of their anatomic defect, if this is indicated.

Patients at the highest risk for complications from an AAA repair are those with a recent myocardial infarction (MI), inoperable CAD, and end-stage pulmonary disease. The treatment options are limited in this group of patients. One may indefinitely defer treatment if the patient's risk appears to be higher than the risk of rupture over the following 2 to 5 years. Alternatively, a "less risky" procedure can be performed (external aneurysm wrapping or an extra-anatomic by-pass with ligation of the aneurysm). However, these techniques do not prevent rupture and are associated with a significant morbidity and mortality. They are of little, if any, value. Proceeding with a conventional AAA repair with an intensive effort to optimize the perioperative condition of the patient is another acceptable alternative. More recently, intraluminal AAA repair is becoming an alternative for these extremely sick patients and may prove to be important to the future of aneurysm surgery.

Patients undergoing elective aneurysm repair should receive a mechanical and antibiotic bowel preparation. Invasive monitoring lines (pulmonary and radial arterial catheters) are placed before the procedure to optimize the patient's hemodynamic status. No antiplatelet or anticoagulant agent should be given for at least 7 days before the elective procedure. Intravenous antibiotics are given on-call to the operating room as prophylaxis against infection.

The operating room must be well equipped for the procedure. The room must be kept warm and a warming blanket should be used to help maintain the patient's body temperature during the procedure. Skin preparation should extend from the chest to the knees to enable full access to the femoral vessels during the procedure. An autotransfusion device is used routinely to minimize the use of homologous blood for transfusion.

The abdominal aorta may be exposed either trans-peritoneally (Fig. 9-3) (midline or transverse incision) or by a retroperitoneal approach. Retroperitoneal exposure through an oblique incision extending from the left eleventh intercostal space to the edge of the rectus abdominis muscle affords excellent aortic exposure; however, the access to the right iliofemoral system is compromised. Factors that favor the use of the retroperitoneal approach include the lack of right iliac artery involvement, obesity, pulmonary disease, and previous abdominal procedures.

The coexistence of other intra-abdominal pathologic conditions that are discovered during abdominal exploration presents specific problems. Malignant tumors (usually colonic) are unexpectedly found in 4% to 5% of patients who undergo elective repair. The aneurysm should be treated as planned unless there are compelling reasons to treat the colonic process first (such as perforation, obstruction, or hemorrhage). Asymptomatic gallstones are found in 5% to 20% of patients. Several series have shown that cholecystectomy at the time of aneurysm repair is safe, but many authors point out the theoretical concern of graft contamination. Tandem atherosclerotic lesions of the aortic branches most often involve the renal arteries in patients with renovascular hypertension or impaired renal function. These can be treated simultaneously; however, the added morbidity and mortality must be considered. Prophylactic procedures should *not* be performed in these situations.

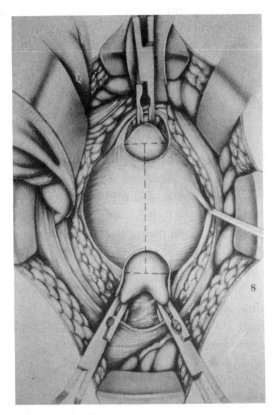

Fig. 9-3. Standard transabdominal approach to the repair of an infrarenal AAA. Arterial control is obtained at the infrarenal aorta and common iliac arteries as shown. The aneurysmal sac is opened along the dotted lines to suture a synthetic graft within the aneurysmal aorta.

Mortality for elective aneurysm repair ranges from 1% to 5%; the higher figure is probably representative of the population at large. The most common cause of death is myocardial dysfunction. Nonfatal MI occurs in 3% to 16% of patients. Excessive hemorrhage may occur intraoperatively or in the immediate postoperative period. When massive bleeding occurs during the operation, it is usually caused by venous injuries (inferior vena cava, iliac, or left renal vein). Postoperative hemorrhage can occur from unrecognized operative injuries or from the anastomoses. Hemodynamic instability and evidence of continued blood loss mandates early surgical reexploration. Renal failure, although infrequent following elective aneurysm repair, is probably caused by reflex renal vasoconstriction, hypovolemia, and intrarenal redistribution of blood flow. Atheromatous debris, temporary suprarenal clamping, and previous renal injury from a large contrast load may be contributing factors. Mannitol is commonly given before aortic cross-clamping in an attempt to prevent these complications.

Gastrointestinal complications are *not* uncommon and range from ileus to colonic infarction. Adynamic ileus is normally present for up to 5 days after surgery. Rarely, a hematoma or edema in the area of the proximal anastomosis will present as a duodenal obstruction in the early postoperative period. Clinical pancreatitis is rare, but postoperative hyperamylasemia is common as a result of pancreatic injury from dissection or retractors. Ischemic colitis is the most serious of these complications, occurring in 2% of patients. The earliest clinical manifestation of bowel ischemia is usually bloody diarrhea. This should prompt an early colono-scopic evaluation of the colonic mucosa. Later findings of peritonitis suggestive of bowel gangrene demand prompt reoperation, removal of the necrotic bowel, and a proximal diverting colostomy. A high index of suspicion is required to diagnose and treat this com-plication as early as possible. Although less severe de-grees of colonic ischemia can be treated nonopera-tively, mortality from this complication approaches 90% when full-thickness gangrene and peritonitis are present.

Lower extremity ischemia is a significant compli-cation following aortic reconstruction. This may be the result of embolization at the time of the repair or thrombosis resulting from blood stasis, an intimal flap, or a crushed atherosclerotic plaque. Administration of heparin should prevent thrombosis caused by stasis during arterial occlusion. Thrombectomy or embo-lectomy may be needed if the distal circulation is com-promised after completion of the aneurysm repair. Microembolization can present with patches of isch-emia at the most distal sites ("trash foot"). Rare com-plications include paraplegia secondary to spinal cord ischemia. This complication is more common after the treatment of a thoracoabdominal aneurysm. In-fection of the prosthetic graft usually presents months to years later with recurrent bacteremia, false aneurysms, intra-abdominal infected collections, or as a graft-enteric fistula.

SPLANCHNIC ARTERY ANEURYSMS

Splenic artery aneurysms account for 60% of all splanchnic aneurysms and are four times more likely to develop in women than in men. Three conditions are associated with the development of these aneurysms: medial fibrodysplasia, increased splenic blood flow (as in cirrhosis or pregnancy), and the effects of increased levels of estrogens on elastic vascular tissue. Other causes are pancreatitis and penetrating trauma. These aneurysms are usually asymptomatic and are found in patients undergoing abdominal evaluations for unrelated symptoms. Epigastric or left upper quadrant pain occurs in up to 20% of patients. The risk of rupture of a splenic aneurysm is 2%, but the surgical mortality after rupture is 25% and may increase to 75% during pregnancy. If intervention is considered necessary in high-risk patients (such as in a pregnant patient or when a splenic aneurysm exceeds 2 cm in maximal diameter), aneurysm embolization may represent a reasonable alternative to decrease the chance of rupture while preserving splenic function. Arterial ligation or excision, splenectomy, or distal pancreatectomy may be necessary in the treatment of this entity.

Hepatic artery aneurysms account for 20% of all splanchnic aneurysms and are twice as likely to develop in men as in women. Conditions associated with the development of these aneurysms include medial degeneration, blunt and penetrating liver trauma, and infection related to intravenous substance abuse. These are usually solitary and extrahepatic (80%). Few are symptomatic, presenting with epigastric or right upper quadrant pain. The risk of rupture of a hepatic aneurysm is 20%, with a surgical mortality after rupture of 35%. These aneurysms have been most often treated with aneurysm resection or exclusion without arterial reconstruction because of the extensive collateral circulation to the liver. In high-risk patients, embolization may be an alternative.

Superior mesenteric artery (SMA) *aneurysms* (Fig. 9-4) account for only 5.5% of all splanchnic aneurysms and have no sex predilection. Conditions associated with their development include: medial degeneration and infection related to bacterial endocarditis and/or intravenous drug abuse. Rupture is uncommon but has an associated mortality of 50%. Thrombosis, although rare, is more common than rupture and will present as acute intestinal ischemia. These aneurysms are treated with aneurysmectomy and SMA reconstruction or ligation if collateral circulation is adequate.

Other splanchnic aneurysms account for the other 12% to 15% of splanchnic aneurysms. They include celiac (4%), gastric and gastroepiploic (4%), jejunal, ileal, or colic (3%), pancreaticoduodenal and pancreat-

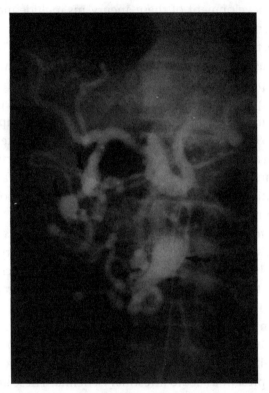

Fig. 9-4. Arteriogram of a patient with multiple mesenteric aneurysms. These include an aneurysm of the superior mesenteric artery (SMA) *(straight arrow)* and two gastroduodenal artery aneurysms *(curved arrows)*.

ic (2%), and gastroduodenal (1.5%) (see Fig. 9-4). These are caused by medial degeneration, connective tissue disorders, and periarterial inflammation (mostly from pancreatitis). The frequency of rupture varies from 13% for celiac aneurysms to up to 90% for gastric and gastroepiploic aneurysms. The associated surgical mortality also varies from 20% for jejunal, ileal, and colic aneurysms to 70% for gastric and gastroepiploic aneurysms. The treatment for these aneurysms is usually surgical: aneurysmectomy with reconstruction or ligation if collateral circulation is adequate for celiac aneurysms; aneurysm excision with associated bowel resection or ligation for gastric, gastroepiploic, jejunal, ileal, colic, pancreaticoduodenal, pancreatic, or gastroduodenal aneurysms. Embolization for specific lesions or high-risk patients has also been used.

Superior Mesenteric Artery Disease

ACUTE MESENTERIC ISCHEMIA. Acute intestinal ischemia can be caused by occlusive (thromboembolic) or nonocclusive disease. The patient typically presents with severe abdominal pain *out of proportion to the* (usually minimal) *physical findings,* marked leukocytosis, and intestinal emptying (diarrhea and vomiting). Later manifestations include bloody stools and diffuse peritonitis, with an associated mortality approaching 100%.

Embolic occlusion is the most common cause of mesenteric occlusion. The triad of abdominal pain, bowel emptying, and a cardiac source of emboli is classic. There are no specific noninvasive tests to diagnose this entity; therefore angiography or laparotomy are needed for diagnosis. Early aortography will delineate the site of occlusion and the existing collateral circulation (Fig. 9-5). The proximal small bowel is usually spared, because the embolus typically lodges distal to the branch of the middle colic artery. This allows perfusion via this vessel as well as through the first few arcades to the proximal small bowel. Embolectomy is performed through an SMA arteriotomy and a mesenteric bypass is constructed if necessary. Assessment of intestinal viability following reestablishment of flow is very difficult. A multitude of techniques have been suggested to aid in determining the extent of bowel resection:

- Inspection (bowel color, motility, pulses or peristalsis)
- Doppler assessment of blood flow to vessels
- Intravenous fluorescein and Wood's lamp investigation
- Oximetry
- Photoplethysmography

Nonviable bowel is resected at the initial operation, but bowel with questionable viability is reassessed within 48 hours and a decision regarding resection is made at the "second-look" operation.

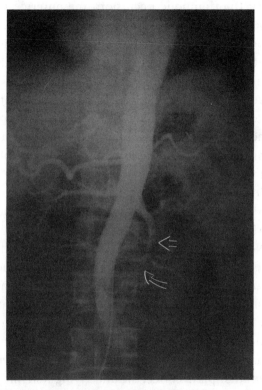

Fig. 9-5. Arteriogram of a patient with sudden onset severe abdominal pain and minimal physical findings 3 days after cardiac surgery. The proximal SMA is partially occluded by an embolus *(straight arrow)* and completely occluded distally *(curved arrow)*.

Mesenteric (SMA) thrombosis. A less common entity than embolic occlusion, mesenteric arterial thrombosis presents with identical clinical manifestations with the important exception of its insidious onset of symptoms. These patients may have a history of chronic intestinal ischemia suggesting disease of the celiac *and* superior mesenteric arteries. Urgent aortography is recommended with selective views of the celiac and SMA arteries. The thrombotic occlusion usually occurs at the site of an arteriosclerotic plaque near the SMA orifice; therefore the ischemic bowel will begin at the ligament of Treitz and extend to the mid-transverse colon. The treatment should include arterial bypass and bowel resection.

Nonocclusive mesenteric ischemia. Nonocclusive mesenteric ischemia is a flow-related phenomenon. It is usually a result of medical conditions such as cardiac failure, cardiac dysrhythmias, myocardial infarction, shock, trauma, aortic valvular insufficiency, or inotropic drugs. The vasoconstrictive response is treated with intra-arterial vasodilators such as papaverine while attempts to correct the underlying systemic problem are undertaken. Angiography is necessary for the diagnosis and treatment of this condition. Findings include a patent mesenteric tree with arterial spasm at different levels. Clinical manifestations are the same as for other conditions leading to mesenteric ischemia. Intra-arterial papaverine, delivered by a catheter in the SMA, is begun when the diagnosis is made angiographically. Laparotomy may be necessary if the patient develops signs of peritonitis.

CHRONIC MESENTERIC ISCHEMIA. The clinical manifestations of chronic mesenteric ischemia include abdominal pain related to meals, occasional diarrhea or constipation, and other signs of generalized atherosclerotic disease (CAD, cerebrovascular disease, or peripheral disease). The combination of weight loss, absence of a carcinoma, and the presence of systemic vascular disease suggests a diagnosis of chronic mesenteric ischemia. Most of these patients have undergone an extensive gastrointestinal workup before this diagnosis is entertained. Endoscopic examinations will all have been noncontributory, as will the multitude of imaging studies. Appropriate diagnostic evaluation should include a duplex scan of the mesenteric circulation, followed by flush lateral aortography and celiac and superior mesenteric selective arteriography. Treatment of chronic mesenteric ischemia is strictly surgical and may include transaortic endarterectomy or visceral artery bypass originating from the aorta or its branches (iliac or hepatic arteries). Autogenous vein or prosthetic material can be used for the bypass. Mesenteric angioplasty can be considered for high-risk patients, but the immediate failure rate is 20%, with a high recurrence rate within a few months. More significantly, acute occlusion resulting from angioplasty complications becomes a surgical emergency with a much less favorable outcome than an elective procedure. We therefore do not recommend balloon angioplasty for any SMA lesions.

Mesenteric Venous Thrombosis

This condition is associated with a previous flu-like syndrome and dehydration. Patients may present with abdominal pain, distention, change in bowel habits and a mild fever. The diagnosis of this condition can now be made with contrast computed tomography and duplex visualization of the portal vein. This condition is often associated with a coagulopathy. A history of previous thrombophlebitis or a family history of venous thrombosis should be sought in these patients. Operative findings in this condition include skip areas of involvement, with bowel edema and engorgement. Anticoagulation therapy is the treatment of choice. Laparotomy should be reserved for patients with signs of peritonitis.

Renal Artery Disease

Occlusive or stenotic lesions of the renal artery can lead to renovascular hypertension and progressive degeneration of renal function. Two distinct causes exist for renal artery occlusive disease: atherosclerosis and *fibromuscular dysplasia* (FMD). Atherosclerotic lesions typically occur at or near the renal artery ostia, are more common on the *left* side and account for 70% of the lesions of renovascular hypertension (Fig. 9-6). FMD represents a constellation of hyperplastic and fibrosing lesions of all layers of the arterial wall. The most common variety, medial fibroplasia, occurs in 70% of cases of FMD and is characterized by an increase in the fibrous connective tissue of the media, with mural aneurysms. Fibromuscular dysplasia is most common in young women. The *right* artery is more often involved than the left but bilateral involvement occurs in the majority of cases. These lesions

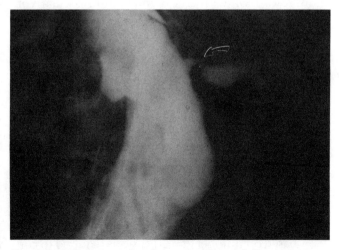

Fig. 9-6. Arteriogram showing a significant left renal artery lesion *(arrow)* with poststenotic dilatation in a patient with worsening renal function and a nonfunctioning right kidney.

have a classic "string of beads" appearance on arteriography.

RENOVASCULAR HYPERTENSION (RVH). Renovascular hypertension has been classified as either renin dependent or volume dependent. Renin-dependent RVH is associated with a *unilateral* renal artery stenosis and a functionally intact contralateral kidney. This allows a rise in renin levels, with subsequent increased amounts of angiotensin II produced. This potent vasoconstrictor will produce systemic hypertension (HTN). When the contralateral renal artery or kidney is diseased, an angiotensin-aldosterone–mediated volume-dependent HTN occurs on the basis of increasing sodium resorption with an expanded intravascular volume.

RVH is likely responsible for approximately 10% of the hypertensive population of patients. However, the appropriate method to screen for RVH in a cost-effective and sensitive manner has yet to be defined. Clinical findings suggestive of the presence of RVH have been suggested:

- Recent onset of hypertension
- Extremes of age (young or old patient)
- Abdominal bruit
- No family history of hypertension
- Severe hypertension (either at presentation or based on number of medications required to control blood pressure)
- Diastolic blood pressure greater than 105 mm Hg

The evaluation of a patient with new onset HTN should be standardized, as shown below:

- Routine blood work (electrolytes, SMA-12, and complete blood count)
- Urine culture
- Electrolytes
- Chest radiograph
- 24-hour urine collection for creatinine clearance
- Catecholamines
- Vanillylmandelic acid
- 17-hydroxysteroids and hydroxyketosteroids
- Intravenous pyelogram
- Renal scan
- Renal angiogram

The rapid-sequence intravenous pyelogram has, generally, been replaced by radionuclide scans which evaluate renal perfusion *and* excretory function. However, these studies continue to have a 25% incidence of false positive and false negative results. The blood pressure response following the administration of a converting-enzyme inhibitor is a simple screening method that is replacing the use of measuring *plasma* renin levels. The lack of a reliable screening test has led many of the more aggressive centers to advocate renal arteriography as a screening tool in patients with a high probability of RVH. Arteriography can be performed with the standard "cut film" technique or with the use of subtraction angiography. Duplex evaluation of the renal artery has promise and may become more widely used as technical expertise increases.

Function tests are valuable in confirming the significance of renal artery stenosis when the contralateral renal artery and kidney are normal; they lose their value when bilateral disease exists. Renal vein renin assays are used to establish a diagnosis of RVH. It is crucial that the test be performed in the following standard fashion to minimize erroneous results:

- One-week salt restriction (2 g sodium diet)
- Discontinuation of all antihypertensive drugs for 5 days (except diuretics)
- Furosemide diuresis (oral) on evening before study
- Bed rest for 4 hours before study

Split renal function studies can also be used to evaluate the significance of arterial lesions. This test is less commonly used because of the associated discomfort, complications, and confusing results.

Patients who should be considered for operative intervention include those with severe or difficult-to-control HTN and young hypertensive patients with no complicating diseases and an easily correctable lesion. In addition, patients with worsening renal function, an atherosclerotic renal artery lesion, and RVH should be considered for operative repair of the renal artery lesion.

Treatment interventions include percutaneous transluminal angioplasty (PTA), aortorenal bypass, ex vivo reconstruction, and thromboendarterectomy. Nephrectomy should be limited to patients with severe

RVH in whom the responsible kidney has unreconstructible vessels with negligible or no residual excretory function and a normal contralateral kidney. Aortorenal bypass is preferentially performed with saphenous vein but can also be done with hypogastric artery or prosthetic material. The hypogastric artery is *preferred* for pediatric reconstructions. Thromboendarterectomy is used only for atherosclerotic renal artery stenosis. PTA can technically be used for any arterial lesion; however, there is a high early failure rate for PTA when performed for atherosclerotic orificial lesions. The results reported for PTA of fibrodysplastic lesions of the main renal artery are similar to those for surgical repairs.

The effects of operation on HTN must be carefully evaluated. Operative mortality has been low ($<1\%$), and a beneficial blood pressure response has been achieved in up to 94% of the patients. Patients with FMD have a much higher chance of cure than those with atherosclerosis (70% to 80% versus 30% to 40%). In addition to these effects, early mortality associated with cardiovascular events may be decreased with improved management of RVH. Renal function can also be improved in a select group of patients who undergo revascularization for worsening azotemia. Only patients with severe renal impairment (creatinine >3.0 mg/dl) and correctable bilateral disease will have a significant improvement in serum creatinine after revascularization.

In summary, PTA of nonorificial atherosclerotic lesions and FMD lesions limited to the main renal artery yields results comparable to that for surgical interventions. Surgery is the treatment of choice for congenital stenotic lesions, FMD lesions involving renal artery branches, and ostial atherosclerotic lesions. The use of renal artery stents is currently being evaluated and shows promise.

BIBLIOGRAPHY

Boley SJ, Brandt LJ, eds. Intestinal ischemia. Surg Clin North Am 72:entire issue, 1992.

Moore WS, ed. Vascular Surgery: A Comprehensive Review, 3rd ed. Philadelphia: WB Saunders, 1991.

Pierce GE, ed. Abdominal aortic aneurysms. Surg Clin North Am 69:entire issue, 1989.

Rutherford RB, ed. Vascular Surgery, 3rd ed. Philadelphia: WB Saunders, 1989.

Veith FJ. Vascular surgical techniques. In Veith FJ, Hobson RW, Williams RA, Wilson SE, eds.Vascular Surgery: Principles and Practice, 2nd ed. New York: McGraw-Hill, 1994, pp 1134-1204.

10

Cerebrovascular Disease

Thomas F. Panetta

The rationale for extracranial cerebrovascular surgical procedures is for prophylaxis of stroke, and less frequently, the treatment of ischemic symptom complexes, including vertebral basilar insufficiency, subclavian steal syndrome, and some cases of flow-related or "watershed" cerebral symptoms. Stroke is the third leading cause of death in the United States. The annual incidence is approximately 195 per 100,000 population, with the highest incidence in elderly males (1440 per 100,000 men, 75 to 84 years old) and the prevalence is approximately 2 million people. The initial mortality of a stroke ranges from 15% to 37%. Survivors have a 6% to 12% risk per year of a metachronous stroke, 35% of which are fatal. Risk factors that increase the relative risk for a stroke include increasing age, male gender, diabetes, and hypertension. An estimated 40% to 75% of patients with ischemic strokes have surgically accessible extracranial carotid and vertebral artery occlusive disease.

Anatomy

The circulation of blood to the brain occurs through the aortic arch vessels and the extracranial and intracranial cerebral vessels. The anatomy is depicted in Figs. 10-1 through 10-3. Embryologically, the carotid arteries originate from the third aortic arch and the dorsal aorta. The carotid bifurcation is usually located at a midcervical level (between C3 and C4), but its location is variable and can range from as high as C1 to as low as T2. Anomalies of the aortic arch include an aberrant right subclavian artery (seen on 0.5% to 1% of arteriograms) originating distal to the left subclavian artery and passing behind the esophagus, and, less commonly, a right aortic arch or double aortic arch. In 10% of cases, the left common carotid artery arises directly from the innominate artery. The vertebral arteries can arise directly from the aorta, from various locations on the subclavian arteries or even from the carotid arteries. The internal carotid artery usually lies posterolateral to the external carotid artery and can be differentiated from the external carotid by the lack of branches in the neck. Kinking or coiling of the internal carotid arteries occurs in 5% to 15% of patients as a result of the disproportionate embryologic migration of the arteries in relation to the spinal cord. Kinking and coiling are usually benign conditions unless associated with significant stenoses, and they are unrelated to either age or hypertension. Congenital absence, hypoplasia, and anomalous branches of the cervical internal carotid artery are rare but reported findings.

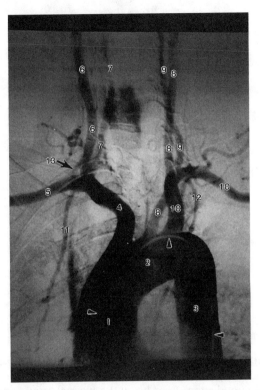

Fig. 10-1. Arch arteriogram. *Arrowheads* point to pigtail catheter in ascending aorta inserted via a transfemoral approach. *1,* Ascending aorta; *2,* aortic arch; *3,* descending aorta; *4,* innominate artery; *5,* right subclavian artery; *6,* right common carotid artery; *7,* right vertebral artery; *8,* left common carotid artery; *9,* left vertebral artery; *10,* left subclavian artery; *11,* right internal mammary artery; *12,* left internal mammary artery; *13,* right thyrocervical trunk.

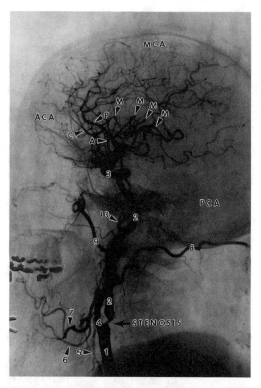

Fig. 10-2. Selected left lateral carotid angiogram. *1,* Common carotid artery; *2,* internal carotid artery; *3,* carotid siphon; *4,* external carotid artery. Branches of the external carotid artery: *5,* superior thyroid artery; *6,* lingual artery; *7,* facial artery; *8,* occipital artery; *9,* maxillary artery; *10,* superficial temporal artery. *A,* Anterior cerebral artery; *C,* callosomarginal artery; *P,* pericallosal artery; *M,* insular branches of the middle cerebral artery; *ACA,* terminal branches of the anterior cerebral artery; *MCA,* terminal branches of the middle cerebral artery; *PCA,* the posterior cerebral artery, which supplies this area, is not shown. A high-grade carotid stenosis is seen at the origin of the internal carotid artery.

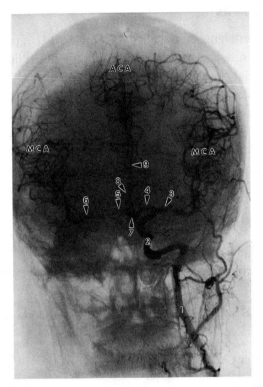

Fig. 10-3. Selected left common carotid artery angiogram. *1,* Internal carotid artery; *2,* carotid siphon; *3,* left middle cerebral artery; *4,* A1 segment of the left anterior cerebral artery; *5,* A1 segment of the right anterior cerebral artery; *6,* right middle cerebral artery; *7,* anterior communicating artery; *8,* right and left A2 segments of anterior cerebral artery; *9,* pericallosal (medial) and callosomarginal (lateral) branches of the anterior cerebral artery; *MCA,* terminal branches of the middle cerebral artery; *ACA,* terminal branches of the anterior cerebral artery.

Diagnosis

The diagnostic classification (Table 10-1) of patients is of paramount importance in defining the indications and relative risks of cerebrovascular surgery. A basic understanding of the pathophysiology of each category is the foundation for developing a therapeutic approach. The majority of symptomatic patients can be classified on the basis of a detailed history and physical examination. Noninvasive testing is performed to screen

Table 10-1. Diagnostic Classification of Patients

Patient Classification	Indications for CEA	Perioperative Risk of CVA
Asymptomatic	Controversial; selected patients	<1%
TIA or amaurosis fugax	Indicated	2% to 4%
Crescendo TIAs	Indicated	2% to 4%
RINDs Stroke (resolved)	Indicated	4% to 6%
Stroke (acute)	Contraindicated	Extremely high risk of hemorrhage
Stroke-in-evolution	Selected patients	Increased
Chronic ischemia	Indicated	<1%
Vertebrobasilar insufficiency	Indicated	<1%

CEA = carotid endarterectomy; CVA = cerebrovascular accident; RINDs = reversible ischemic neurologic deficits; TIAs = transient ischemic attacks.

patients and confirm the clinical suspicion of carotid stenosis. The use of CT or magnetic resonance imaging (MRI) of the head to document strokes in symptomatic and asymptomatic patients is necessary for a definitive classification.

An *asymptomatic carotid stenosis* is defined as any preocclusive atherosclerotic plaque in the common carotid artery, the carotid bifurcation, or the internal carotid artery in a patient with no ipsilateral monocular or cerebral hemispheric symptoms. Acute neurologic deficits are differentiated as *transient ischemic attacks* (TIAs) or strokes based on whether the focal deficit resolves within or persists longer than 24 hours, respectively. Approximately 75% of patients with strokes have had previous TIAs. *Amaurosis fugax* is defined as transient monocular blindness caused by embolic central retinal artery occlusion or retinal cholesterol emboli (Hollenhorst plaque). A *stroke-in-evolution* differs from a stroke in that after the initial neurologic event, symptoms wax and wane, with progression rather than resolution. *Reversible ischemic neurologic deficits* (RINDs) persist for longer than 24 hours but resolve within 72 hours. *Crescendo TIAs* are monocular or hemispheric symptoms that resolve within minutes after each episode but increase in frequency, occurring several times a day. Patients categorized as having *chronic cerebral ischemia* are those with multiple, extracranial, cerebrovascular arterial occlusions who have nonspecific or global cerebral ischemic symptoms. These symptoms include lightheadedness, presyncope, ataxia, or even the subjective impression of compromised cerebral function. ***Vertebrobasilar system TIAs*** manifest any combination of motor dysfunction, sensory loss, homonymous visual field deficits, and posterior circulation symptoms (loss of balance, vertigo, dysequilibrium, diplopia, dysarthria, or dysphagia).

The relative risk of stroke or blindness in any patient is a multifactorial problem related to the patient's symptom status (asymptomatic, TIA, previous stroke), the severity of the carotid stenosis, and the type of disease (soft plaque, calcification, hemorrhage) within the carotid artery. In addition to the increased risk associated with intrinsic carotid bifurcation disease, systemic factors such as hypertension, diabetes, cardiac disease, smoking, and reduced levels of high density lipoproteins play a role.

Evaluation of the patient with cerebrovascular disease includes a complete history, a neurologic examination, and an evaluation of related vascular and cerebral pathology. A careful history will usually establish both the location and severity of the cerebral event in addition to suggesting the pathophysiologic mechanism. Neurological symptoms resulting from ischemic events in a particular area of the brain are evaluated to determine whether they are causally related to embolic events in the vascular territory supplying that portion of the brain. Rather than discussing a generic neurologic examination, symptom complexes will be related to the anatomic patterns of emboli correlating the end organ with the vascular supply.

MIDDLE CEREBRAL ARTERY. The middle cerebral artery is the largest branch of the internal carotid artery and the artery most often involved in TIAs and stroke. Large infarcts involve the cortex, basal ganglia, and internal capsule, resulting in contralateral hemiplegia, global aphasia when the dominant hemisphere is involved, head and eye deviation toward the side of the infarct, hemianesthesia, and hemianopsia (hemineglect of the opposite side).

Middle cerebral artery (upper division). The middle cerebral artery is the most common area affected by TIAs manifest by contralateral hemiparesis and hemianesthesia of the face and arm (more than the leg), motor aphasia (Broca's) when the dominant hemisphere is involved, and hemianopsia.

Middle cerebral artery (lower division). Aphasia and hemianopsia in the absence of hemiparesis occur when the dominant hemisphere is involved. When the nondominant hemisphere is involved, hemianopsia and behavior disturbances are the only manifestations.

Middle cerebral artery (penetrating lenticulostriate arteries). These lenticulostriate arteries supply the internal capsule, resulting in a lacunar infarct (descriptive of the cavitary pathologic appearance) manifest by pure hemiparesis without sensory loss, aphasia, or visual or behavioral abnormalities. Other symptom complexes include pure sensory stroke, ataxic hemiparesis, or the dysarthria–clumsy hand syndrome. In patients with these strokes, imaging studies of the brain may yield normal results.

ANTERIOR CEREBRAL ARTERY. Since this artery supplies the paracentral lobule, infarction or TIAs manifest motor and sensory loss of the contralateral leg (distal greater than proximal). Contralateral proximal arm weakness, discriminative sensory loss, tactile anomia, clumsiness, apraxia, and agraphia can occur.

POSTERIOR CEREBRAL ARTERY. The posterior cerebral artery is the terminal branch of the basilar artery; it supplies the temporal and occipital lobes. As part of the posterior circulation, it is less frequently affected by embolization. However, emboli from the internal carotid artery can reach the posterior circulation through the posterior communicating arteries. Visual field deficits or hemianopsia can result from occipital cortex involvement. Symptom complexes related to midbrain and thalamic infarcts include third nerve palsies, hemiplegia, hypesthesia or sensory loss, Horner's syndrome, memory disturbances, obtundation, and stupor.

VERTEBROBASILAR ARTERIES. Symptoms referable to the posterior circulation are usually related to multiple occlusions, resulting in hemodynamic disturbances and, rarely, in emboli. Physical examination should include bilateral blood pressure measurements to identify hemodynamically significant proximal subclavian or innominate disease. Symptoms of vertebrobasilar insufficiency (VBI) include dizziness or vertigo; occipital headache; visual disturbances caused by diplopia, ataxia, dysphagia, and nausea and vomiting; perioral numbness; and facial paralysis. TIAs have been reported in 5% to 30% of patients with VBI. Symptoms referable to the middle cerebral artery (hemiparesis and aphasia) can occur in patients with combined carotid and vertebral occlusive disease, an absent anterior communicating artery and a patent posterior communicating artery which steals blood from the anterior circulation.

Subclavian steal syndrome is a specific pathophysiologic and anatomic complex that leads to reversal of blood flow in the vertebral artery as a result of a proximal subclavian or innominate artery occlusion. It is more common on the left than on the right side, since the left subclavian is an isolated artery and does not communicate with the carotid. Therefore the anatomy of the innominate artery is protective. Arm ischemia is rare in these patients, although a significant difference in blood pressure frequently exists between the two arms. A decreased radial artery pulse in conjunction with symptoms of VBI exacerbated by arm exercise is pathognomonic. The diagnosis is confirmed

angiographically by late films demonstrating filling
of the distal subclavian by retrograde vertebral blood
flow (Fig. 10-4) or duplex ultrasonographic detection
of reversal of blood flow in the vertebral artery.

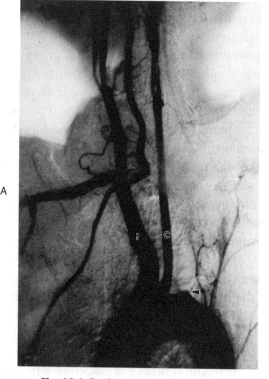

Fig. 10-4. For legend see opposite page.

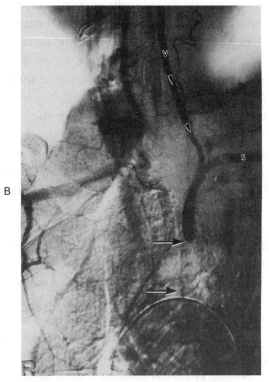

Fig. 10-4. A, Arteriogram of a patient with subclavian steal syndrome. *I,* innominate artery; *C,* left carotid artery. *Arrowhead* points to the origin of the occlusion in the left subclavian artery which is not shown. **B,** Delayed arteriogram demonstrating retrograde visualization of the left vertebral *(V)* and left subclavian *(S)* arteries. *Arrowheads* depict reversal of flow in the vertebral artery; *large black arrows* demonstrate length of the proximal subclavian artery occlusion.

Physical examination. Physical examination of the extracranial circulation includes palpation of common carotid, internal carotid, and temporal artery pulsations. Before auscultation of the carotids and vertebrals for the presence of bruits is done, precordial auscultation should be performed to determine the presence of cardiac murmurs, especially aortic ejection murmurs, which can be transmitted up the carotid arteries. The examiner should be able to document a decrease in intensity of cardiac murmurs as one moves up the neck, with a concomitant increase in the intensity of carotid bruits. Another differentiating feature is that carotid bruits extend into diastole as a result of the low peripheral resistance of the cerebral circulation. Auscultation for systolic and early diastolic bruits should be performed above and below the sternoclavicular joints (vertebral and subclavian bruits) and in the lower third, middle third and upper third of the neck just anterior to the border of the sternomastoid muscle. Bruits become manifest with a 50% reduction in arterial diameter (a 75% reduction in cross sectional area of the artery = πr^2) which represents a hemodynamically significant stenosis. As the stenosis increases above 95%, the bruit may disappear as the blood flow diminishes. The sudden disappearance of a bruit (for example, during an arteriogram) is considered diagnostic of carotid occlusion and is an indication for emergent carotid endarterectomy.

Hollenhorst, an ophthalmologist at the Mayo Clinic, first described cholesterol crystals as bright yellowish material in the retinal arteries discovered on ophthalmoscopic examination of patients with amaurosis fugax. The finding of Hollenhorst plaques may not be temporally related to the symptoms of amaurosis fugax, but they are pathognomonic for emboli from the carotid arteries rather than the heart. Amaurosis fugax in the absence of Hollenhorst plaques can be caused by platelet-fibrin complexes (sometimes visualized as pale, white or grayish material migrating at the time of symptoms) that dissipate, emboli in the choroidal circulation that are not visualized on ophthalmoscopic examination, or the presence of low-flow states resulting in symptoms. White, nonscintillating calcific emboli and pallor of the disc have also been reported. The finding of a Hollenhorst plaque is associated with all forms of cerebrovascular disease (not just amaurosis fugax), and it is a marker for both systemic atherosclerosis and atherosclerotic coronary artery disease. Its presence is not associated with an increased risk of retinal infarction, although as a group, patients with amaurosis fugax do have an increased incidence of ischemic optic neuropathy, resulting in visual loss and even blindness.

Other diagnostic measures. *Duplex ultrasonography* is the gold standard procedure for the noninvasive diagnosis of the extracranial cerebrovascular circulation. This test incorporates B-mode ultrasono-graphic imaging techniques with spectral frequency analysis of pulsed-Doppler signals. The degree of stenosis is determined by a combination of the degree of elevation of the peak systolic velocity and the amount of spectral broadening. Table 10-2 characterizes flow velocities and spectral broadening to determine the degree of internal carotid artery stenosis. Frequency and velocity data are recorded using a 5 MHz Doppler carrier frequency at a 60-degree angle of insonation. In the hands of experienced technicians, duplex ultra-

Table 10-2. Duplex Ultrasonography Criteria

Diameter Reduction (%)	Peak Systole (cm/sec)	End Diastole (cm/sec)	Flow Character
0	<125	—	No spectral broadening
1 to 15	<125	—	Minimal spectral broadening
16 to 49	<125	—	Increased spectral broadening
50 to 79	>125	—	Marked spectral broadening
80 to 99	>125	>140	Marked spectral broadening
Total occlusion	N/A	N/A	No flow signal

N/A = no flow detected.

sonography demonstrates approximately 95% to 99% sensitivity for determining stenosis. However, it is difficult to differentiate between total occlusions and extremely high-grade stenoses ("string sign") using this test. Color duplex facilitates the technical aspects of performing these studies but adds very little to the overall accuracy. B-mode imaging is useful for determining ulceration, plaque morphology, and the presence of calcification, clot, and hemorrhage. Accessible arteries include the common carotid above the clavicle to the internal carotid below the angle of the mandible, the external carotid artery, and the proximal vertebral arteries.

Duplex ultrasonography is indicated as a screening test for both symptomatic and asymptomatic patients suspected of having extracranial cerebrovascular occlusive disease. This includes all patients with carotid bruits, symptomatic patients without carotid bruits, postoperative follow-up after carotid endarterectomy, serial examinations to follow progression of disease, and screening for vertebrobasilar insufficiency.

Oculoplethysmography (OPG-Gee or oculopneumoplethysmography) involves transduced measurements of ophthalmic artery pressures. It is an accurate technique for identifying hemodynamically significant carotid artery stenosis. However, this test has been supplanted by the more accurate duplex ultrasonography, and it is no longer required for the noninvasive evaluation of the extracranial carotid circulation.

Transcranial Doppler (TCD) uses pulsed-Doppler techniques that allow penetration of "windows" within the skull and has a large enough sample size to permit evaluation of the intracranial cerebral circulation. Blood flow velocities are determined for specific arteries based on the angle and location of the probe, the depth of penetration and the direction and characteristics of the velocities. The arteries accessible to the TCD include the middle cerebral arteries (MCA), the anterior cerebral arteries (ACA), the posterior cerebral arteries (PCA), the internal carotid arteries (parasellar, genu, supraclinoid), the ophthalmic arteries, the vertebral arteries, and the basilar artery. With appropriate compression of carotid arteries, the status of the anterior and posterior communicating arteries and the presence of collaterals between the external carotid and internal carotid arteries (reversal of flow in the ophthalmic artery) can be determined. Peak velocities are greatest in the MCA and lowest in the PCA.

The TCD is useful for the preoperative screening of patients with suspected intracranial occlusive disease, defining the collateral circulation in the circle of Willis and continuous intraoperative monitoring of patients undergoing carotid endarterectomy. During intraoperative monitoring, continuous recording of the MCA velocities are performed. A 60% reduction in mean velocity during clamping is an indication of the need for a shunt.

Computed tomography (CT) of the head is useful in identifying silent infarcts, determining the timing of surgery, evaluating the risk of surgery and ruling out other causes of disease. The first phase of edema occurs 24 to 48 hours after a cerebral infarct, but it can be detected at 6 hours by CT. Contrast enhancement is not necessary to visualize these changes, and because of the potential toxicity of the contrast medium in the area of the infarct, noncontrast CT scans should be performed initially, especially in symptomatic patients. The second phase of an infarct involves macrophage invasion and proliferation of capillaries and occurs in the second to third week after the infarct. During this phase, the infarct may become isodense, resulting in "fogging" or poor visualization on noncontrast enhanced CT scans. The third phase is the result of glial scar and cyst formation that is, again, prominent on noncontrast CT scans. Early on, contrast can also mask acute hemorrhage, which can be visualized before organization (after 24 to 48 hours) on noncontrast CT scans. Although MRI has been shown to be more sensitive than CT scans for determining cerebral infarction, the lack of access to an MRI in many hospitals probably accounts for the continued use of CT scanning over MRI for preoperative screening of patients undergoing carotid endarterectomy.

A complete workup of the patient being considered for cerebral arteriography and carotid endarterectomy includes pertinent laboratory data to evaluate coagulation and viscosity factors (CBC, platelets, PT, PTT, fibrinogen) and to consider the possibility of arteritis, especially when atypical visual symptoms are present (erythrocyte sedimentation rate). Cardiac evaluation for a potential source of cerebral emboli includes an ECG, echocardiography, and a Holter monitor examination. In cases of vertebrobasilar insufficiency, electronystagmography should be performed to rule out the possibility that middle ear disease is a contributing factor.

As with all peripheral vascular diseases, the presence of cerebrovascular disease is a marker for atherosclerotic cardiovascular disease, the major reason for perioperative and long-term mortality in this group of patients. A complete workup for the presence of myocardial disease is mandatory and should include preoperative dipyridamole-thallium stress testing in selected patients. In patients with an increased risk of myocardial infarction, consideration should be given to performing carotid endarterectomy with local anesthesia.

Preoperative radiographic imaging of the arch vessels, the extracranial cerebral vasculature and intracranial circulation is the standard of care in patients considered for carotid endarterectomy. Arteriography is the gold standard and is still our preferred method of preoperative assessment of arterial anatomy and pathology, although the reported complications of stroke and death range from 0.2% to 0.7%. Noninvasive modalities, such as magnetic resonance angiography, combined duplex ultrasonography and transcranial Doppler, or duplex ultrasonography alone, are attractive because they avoid the contrast- and catheter-related complications associated with arteriography. However, in our practice, we use these modalities in lieu of arteriography only in selected cases, particularly in patients with a history of serious contrast reactions.

Arteriography includes complete assessment of the aortic arch as well as selected injections of individual carotid and subclavian arteries with anteroposterior, lateral, and oblique views to evaluate all of the intracranial and extracranial cerebral arteries. Oblique views are necessary to visualize the origins of both vertebral arteries. When done correctly, standard arteriography is the most accurate preoperative study and it affords the most information, including the diagnosis of occlusive, stenotic, or ulcerative cerebrovascular disease; the status of the circle of Willis; visualization of collaterals, which confirms the diagnosis of significant occlusive disease; the diagnosis of steal syndromes (for example, late retrograde filling of the vertebral artery supplying a subclavian artery distal to a proximal occlusion); and the differential diagnosis of trauma (intimal flaps, pseudoaneurysms, arteriovenous fistulas), dissection and arteritis.

Intra-arterial digital subtraction arteriography (DSA) and magnetic resonance arteriography (MRA) are useful in selected cases. Although they are advantageous in that DSA reduces the contrast load and MRA eliminates it, DSA tends to underestimate and MRA overestimate the degree of carotid occlusive disease.

Indications for Carotid Endarterectomy

Although many of the indications remain controversial, the North America Symptomatic Carotid Endarterectomy Trial (NASCET) has clearly demonstrated the benefits of carotid endarterectomy over medical management in patients with high-grade stenosis ($\geq$70%) who are symptomatic (TIA, amaurosis fugax, or previous stroke). The benefits of carotid endarterectomy over medical management became apparent within 3 months of surgery. Carotid endarterectomy reduced the risk of an ipsilateral stroke within 2 years by 17% (medical management versus surgery, 29% and 9%, respectively). The risk of a major or fatal ipsilateral stroke was reduced from 13.1% for the medically treated patients to 2.5% for the surgically treated patients. Likewise, the risk of TIAs, any stroke, or death for up to 30 months of follow-up was reduced by carotid endarterectomy.

Although the national and international trials regarding symptomatic patients with <70% carotid stenoses are not yet completed, it is clear that carefully selected patients benefit from carotid endarterectomy. Consideration should be given to the patient's age, medical risk factors, frequency and nature of symptoms (for example, clear-cut TIA versus vague symptoms), anticipated surgical results, and confidence in accuracy of preoperative tests. For example, biplane arteriography can underestimate the degree of atheromatous debris within the carotid bifurcation. Occasionally duplex ultrasonography will demonstrate a hemodynamically significant high-grade lesion (for example, increased peak systolic velocities) in the patient with <70% stenosis as demonstrated by arteriography.

Asymptomatic carotid stenosis remains a relative indication for carotid endarterectomy. The Veterans Administration (VA) Cooperative Clinical Trial demonstrated better outcome (reduced neurological "events" including TIAs) for surgically versus medically treated patients. However, in the VA study, overall reduction of stroke and death as a result of surgery did not reach statistical significance. The operative mortality (4 fatal MIs = 1.9%) in this study points out the importance of perioperative cardiovascular risk factors and suggests a role for local/regional anesthesia or careful anesthetic management in high-risk patients.

An asymptomatic patient with a carotid bruit should undergo duplex ultrasonography and a CT scan of the head. An unsuspected stroke discovered on the CT scan could reclassify the carotid lesion as symptomatic. Duplex ultrasonography provides important information on the degree of stenosis, the status of the contralateral carotid, the status of the vertebral arteries, and the rate of progression on serial studies. Selected asymptomatic patients with high-grade carotid stenosis should be considered for carotid endarterectomy if they are a good operative risk and have bilateral disease, progression of disease on serial duplex scans, or a contralateral occlusion. Arteriography may be helpful in equivocal cases to identify the status of collaterals, the patency of anterior and posterior communicating arteries, and the extent of extracranial and intracranial occlusive disease.

Patients with combined symptomatic coronary artery occlusive disease requiring coronary artery bypass who have concurrent symptomatic or asymptomatic carotid disease pose a problem: combined carotid endarterectomy and coronary artery bypass is associated with increased morbidity and mortality. Recent evidence suggests, however, that with asymptomatic carotid stenosis, the perioperative stroke rate is decreased by the anticoagulation therapy used during coronary artery bypass. This protective effect allows coronary bypass and subsequent endarterectomy if indicated. In patients with symptomatic carotid disease, consideration should be given to performing carotid endarterectomy under regional/local anesthesia before coronary artery bypass grafting.

The chief contraindication for carotid endarterectomy is the presence of an acute stroke. Revascularization of an acute stroke dramatically increases the risk of hemorrhage into the infarct. Several descriptions in the early literature of the disastrous consequences of hemorrhagic cerebral infarction following carotid endarterectomy in this setting led to a policy of avoiding carotid endarterectomy in an acutely symptomatic patient for up to 2 weeks at a minimum after the onset of symptoms. Exceptions to this rule include some cases of stroke-in-evolution, trauma, select patients in whom carotid endarterectomy can be performed within 6 hours of the onset of symptoms, or patients who have minimal, residual neurologic deficits and a negative CT scan of the head. One example of this is a patient who loses a preexisting bruit and develops symptoms of an infarct at the time of arteriography. Immediate endarterectomy can be successful in restoring the patient's baseline neurologic status. In the trauma setting, coma is the contraindication for carotid revascularization. Short of unresponsiveness, patients with carotid injuries and dense neurologic deficits should undergo a revascularization procedure.

Anesthesia and Monitoring

The controversy about the type of anesthesia (local with or without regional block versus general anesthesia), the method of intraoperative monitoring (awake neurologic status, stump pressure, electroencephalography, somatosensory evoked potentials, transcranial Doppler, or cerebral blood flow) and need for shunting (never shunting, selectively shunting, and routinely shunting) are integrally related. There are reports in the literature demonstrating excellent results using each of these modalities. Each monitoring technique is founded on its ability to detect critical cerebral ischemia resulting from inadequate collateral circulation through the circle of Willis during carotid cross-clamping.

Cerebral ischemia has been estimated to occur in 4% to 33% of patients undergoing carotid endarterectomy. These percentages combine ischemia caused by intraoperative embolic events, which is more common, and ischemia caused by inadequate regional cerebral blood flow, which is less common but requires intraoperative shunting. Flow-related cerebral ischemia would probably occur in only 4% to 6% of cases without the use of a shunt. This incidence increases to as high as 12% to 25% in patients with a contralateral carotid artery occlusion. Intraoperative embolic events can be reduced only by meticulous attention to intraoperative details and faultless operative technique.

The use of local anesthesia permits intraoperative monitoring of the neurologic status of a sedated patient. Patients are selectively shunted if loss of consciousness or loss of upper extremity motor activity (monitored by the ability to squeeze an object that produces a sound) occurs after carotid artery clamping. Regional cervical block can be used as an adjunctive procedure, but it carries the risk of injury to the carotid artery. The use of local anesthesia has distinct advantages, including decreased risk of perioperative myocardial infarction, less blood pressure fluctuations, and decreased ICU stay. The disadvantages include patients who develop agitation and, rarely, seizures during the procedure. These patients require conversion to a general anesthetic.

General anesthesia is thought to impart a protective effect on the brain during periods of ischemia. Although the ability to monitor the awake patient is lost, alternative monitoring techniques with improved thresholds for determining ischemia are used in anesthetized patients. The relative thresholds for monitoring techniques are correlated with cerebral blood flow in Fig. 10-5, which depicts the relationship between the severity and duration of cerebral ischemia. The critical level of cerebral ischemia is at a cerebral blood flow of approximately 15 ml/100 g of brain/min. Intraoperative xenon cerebral blood flow monitoring is extremely accurate, but it is costly, cumbersome, and available only in select centers performing investigational studies. The methods of intraoperative monitoring described next attempt to identify a "window" for detection of cerebral ischemia or inadequate blood flow before the onset of membrane permeability changes and the ultimate development of irreversible neurologic damage.

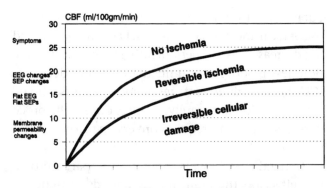

Fig. 10-5. The relationship between duration of ischemia, severity of ischemia, symptoms, thresholds for monitoring techniques and membrane permeability changes. (From Panetta TF, Legatt AD, Veith FJ. Somatosensory Evoked Potential Monitoring During Carotid Surgery. In Greenhalgh RM, Hollier LH, eds. Surgery for Stroke. London: WB Saunders Ltd, 1993, p 275.)

Stump pressure, a measurement of the mean arterial back pressure in the internal carotid artery that is clamped proximally, is a valid and simple method for determining the need for a shunt. Care should be taken to temporarily occlude the internal carotid artery above the measuring site to demonstrate a flat tracing, thus documenting that the measurement is a true stump pressure and not that of an unoccluded branch of the external carotid artery. Patients with stump pressures of less than 25 mm Hg require shunting.

With ***intraoperative electroencephalography,*** a 50% or greater increase in theta or delta activity or a decrease in alpha or beta activity is an indication of cerebral ischemia. Although this technique is widely used, it remains more subjective and has a slightly higher false positive rate than somatosensory evoked potential monitoring.

We prefer the use of ***somatosensory evoked potential*** (SEP) monitoring to determine the degree of cerebral ischemia during carotid artery clamping so that we can selectively shunt. The use of SEPs during carotid surgery is based on the fact that ascending pathways to the thalamus and cortex that receive sensory input after stimulation of the median nerve are supplied by branches of the internal carotid artery (lenticulostriate and middle cerebral). Reduced cerebral blood flow to critical levels during carotid clamping is manifest by a 50% or greater reduction in the amplitude of the N20 waveform (N = negative waveform; 20 = 20 msec of latency), which indicates the need for a shunt. This modality can be used to shunt all patients selectively, including those with a previous stroke or contralateral carotid occlusion.

Transcranial Doppler evaluation is used to determine waveforms and peak systolic velocities in the intracranial arteries, collateral arteries, and the circle of Willis. During carotid endarterectomy, continuous monitoring of the Doppler signal from the middle cerebral artery provides an index of cerebral blood flow during carotid clamping. A decrease in the mean velocity to less than 30 cm/sec is indicative of decreased flow and indicates the need for a shunt. TCD is also useful in identifying microembolic events (most of which are subclinical) that occur at the time of carotid unclamping.

In lieu of monitoring during carotid surgery, many prefer the use of routine shunting in all cases. However, shunts can clot, dislodge, create distal, intimal flaps, and generally make the endarterectomy more difficult to perform. Although these problems are rare, shunts can increase the clamp time required for meticulous endarterectomy and patching.

Surgical Considerations

Carotid endarterectomy is performed with the patient in the supine position, the table flexed, a pillow under the knees, the table in reverse Trendelenburg position (to empty the neck veins), with the table rotated away from the operating surgeon (to facilitate the assistant's role). Carotid endarterectomy is performed in the deep plane of the external elastic lamina. Patching has been shown to be beneficial in patients with small internal carotid arteries and in women. However, as with shunting, there are three different philosophies in regard to patching: routine patching, selective patching (small arteries or women), or non-patching (routine primary closure). Neck wounds are closed in at least three layers with interrupted absorbable sutures. The use of a drain also depends on the surgeon's preference.

The issue of carotid patching, like intraoperative shunting, can be divided into three categories based on individual surgeons' philosophies. Selective patching is performed for small diameter carotid arteries (<3 mm diameter internal carotid artery). Additional indications for some surgeons include whether the patient is a woman, has a hypercoagulable state, or has recurrent stenosis. The greater saphenous vein from the groin is the patch material of choice. Saphenous vein harvested from the ankle is associated with an increased risk of vein patch rupture. Synthetic patches, especially polytetrafluoroethylene (PTFE), provide comparable results, but have the disadvantage of increased needle hole bleeding. We prefer the use of PTFE patches in cases in which an anticipated bypass (for example, aortofemoral, femoropopliteal, femorofemoral) will be needed in the immediate future. There is increasing evidence that improved short- and long-term results are obtained with the use of either routine or selective patching.

Carotid endarterectomy is associated with both intraoperative and postoperative blood pressure fluctuations. Although these fluctuations usually disappear within 48 hours after surgery, strict attention to perioperative blood pressure control is imperative to reduce the operative risk of stroke. These fluctuations in blood pressure are a multifactorial problem and have been related to general anesthesia, cerebral "dysautoregulation," diabetes, carotid sinus nerve stimulation, changes in adventitial stretching following removal of the plaque, cerebral ischemia, cerebral edema, and a variety of vasoactive neurochemical metabolites (such as catecholamines, dopamine, and renins). Tight control of blood pressure (systolic pressure between 120 and 180 mm Hg) during the perioperative period can be achieved by intraoperative carotid sinus nerve injection with lidocaine *or* intravenous neosynephrine for hypotension and nitroglycerine or nitroprusside for hypertension.

Postoperative Care

Postoperative evaluation includes neurologic monitoring for complications and stroke. Patients with postoperative focal neurologic deficits require documentation of carotid artery patency by either duplex ultrasonography and/or operative exploration. Nonstroke complications of carotid endarterectomy include cranial nerve injury, hyperperfusion syndromes (migraines, vasodilatation, inappropriate ADH syndrome, and psychiatric disturbances), intracranial hemorrhage, and cerebral edema. CT scanning and repeat arteriography demonstrating arterial dilatation are useful for the diagnosis and management of these syndromes.

Antiplatelet therapy is the mainstay of therapy in both the surgically and medically treated patient. Patients undergoing carotid endarterectomy should receive aspirin preoperatively and immediately postoperatively as well as heparin intraoperatively. Intraoperative and postoperative administration of dextran is useful, especially in difficult cases (for example, high endarterectomy, small arteries). Dipyridamole is prescribed for at least 3 months after surgery to allow endothelialization of the endarterectomized artery. Thereafter, only the aspirin is continued for life. Low-dose aspirin (65 mg/day) is utilized to inhibit thromboxane synthetase in platelets while preserving prostacyclin synthetase in endothelial cells. The combination of antiplatelet and anticoagulant therapy reduces the risk of perioperative carotid occlusion and stroke but increases the risk of bleeding complications, including wound hematomas. The use of drains is based on the surgeon's preference. With or without the use of drains, antiplatelet agents increase the rate of return to the operating room for evacuation of hematoma, and the patient should be watched closely and be informed of the risk.

The incidence of recurrent carotid stenosis varies, depending on the method of patient evaluation. Symptomatic recurrent stenosis occurs in 1% to 4% of patients, with asymptomatic stenosis occurring much more frequently. Remodeling and subsequent regression of intimal hyperplastic lesions are thought to occur in the majority of asymptomatic stenoses; these cases should be monitored by repeated duplex ultrasonography. Progression of disease to a high-grade stenosis or the development of symptoms are indications for repeat surgical intervention. Because of the high incidence of subsequent recurrences, replacement of the carotid by a saphenous vein bypass is preferred for both early disease (intimal hyperplasia occurring less than 2 years postoperatively) or recurrent atherosclerosis (more than 2 years postoperatively by definition).

Vertebrobasilar Disease

Vertebral artery surgery composes from 2% to 5% of operations for extracranial cerebrovascular occlusive disease. Whereas carotid artery disease, which causes stroke, is chiefly caused by embolic disease, symptoms of vertebrobasilar insufficiency (VBI) are caused by reduced blood flow. The cause of VBI, therefore, includes bilateral vertebral artery stenoses or occlusion or subclavian steal syndrome. Symptoms of VBI include vertigo, ataxia, paresis, numbness, dysphagia, dysarthria, and diplopia. Approximately 5% of patients with VBI present with TIAs because of the hemodynamic stealing of blood from the middle cerebral artery circulation. The majority of these patients have combined vertebral and carotid artery occlusive disease.

The diagnosis is confirmed by duplex ultrasonography and arteriography. Arteriography must include selected subclavian injections with oblique views to identify stenoses at the origins of the vertebral arteries. Standard arteriographic views do not allow visualization of the origins of the vertebral arteries, which are posterior to and obscured by the anterior subclavian arteries.

The treatment of VBI consists of increasing the blood flow to the posterior circulation. In approximately 85% of patients, this can be accomplished by carotid endarterectomy. Selected patients are candidates for direct vertebral artery reconstruction. Direct transposition of the vertebral artery to the carotid artery is the procedure of choice for proximal vertebral artery lesions in the absence of proximal carotid artery disease.

The components of subclavian steal syndrome include a lesion proximal to the vertebral artery (subclavian or innominate) and reversal of flow in the vertebral artery (usually with arm exercise, but it can occur at rest). Arm ischemia is rare, even with total occlusion of the subclavian artery. The treatment is a carotid-subclavian bypass, which is free of the risk of steal from the carotid circulation when there is no proximal carotid lesion. Usually this bypass procedure is performed with a prosthetic graft. This approach not only avoids a thoracotomy but allows the performance of a carotid endarterectomy in the same setting.

EC-IC Bypass

The use of an extracranial-intracranial (EC-IC) bypass has fallen into disfavor for the treatment of extracranial cerebrovascular occlusive disease because of the relatively high perioperative stroke and morbidity rates. An EC-IC bypass involves a direct approach to the intracranial arteries through a craniotomy. The bypass utilizes branches of the external carotid artery or vein grafts originating from branches of the external or common carotid arteries. The bypasses are routed through subcutaneous tunnels anterior to the ear. EC-IC bypasses may still play a role in the treatment of trauma as well as intracranial pathologic conditions such as aneurysms, arteriovenous malformations, moyamoya disease, low perfusion syndrome, and tumors. However, in symptomatic patients with internal carotid artery (ICA) occlusion, consideration should be given to performing an ipsilateral external carotid artery endarterectomy with exclusion of the cul-de-sac in the ICA, a contralateral carotid endarterectomy, or vertebral transposition, depending on the arterial pathology.

BIBLIOGRAPHY

Greenhalgh RM, Hollier LH, eds. Surgery for Stroke. London: WB Saunders Ltd, 1993.

Hobson RW II, Weiss DG, Fields WS, Goldstone J, Moore WS, Towne JB, Wright CB, Veterans Affairs Cooperative Study Group. Efficacy of carotid endarterectomy for asymptomatic carotid stenosis. N Engl J Med 328:221-279, 1993.

North American Symptomatic Carotid Endarterectomy Trial Collaborators. Beneficial effect of carotid endarterectomy in symptomatic patients with high-grade carotid stenosis. N Engl J Med 325:445-507, 1991.

Rosenberg N. Monitoring and use of a shunt during carotid surgery. In CRC Handbook of Carotid Artery Surgery: Facts and Figures. Boca Raton, Fla: CRC Press, 1989, pp 151-170.

11

Vascular Emergencies

Clifford M. Sales • Jamie Goldsmith • Frank J. Veith

The vascular emergencies addressed in this chapter range in scope from the diabetic foot infection to disruption of the abdominal aorta. Although the magnitude of these entities may appear to be distinct, they all mandate early recognition and rapid institution of appropriate therapy.

Ruptured Abdominal Aortic Aneurysm

DIAGNOSIS

History and physical examination. An untreated *ruptured abdominal aortic aneurysm* (RAAA) has a mortality of 100%. The diagnosis must be made *solely* by history and physical examination without the aid of more sophisticated diagnostic tests. The triad of abdominal pain, syncope, and a pulsatile abdominal mass is nearly pathognomonic for a RAAA (Table 11-1). If this triad, or a variation thereof, is present, *no* further diagnostic tests should be performed and the patient must be transported, *without delay,* to the operating room. These patients are often triaged by personnel who are unaware of the triad and at a time that is remote from the patient's initial hypotensive episode.

Table 11-1. Clinical Diagnosis of Ruptured Abdominal Aortic Aneurysm

Classic Presentation	Common Variants
Abdominal pain	Back pain
	Groin pain
	Flank pain
Syncope	Hypotension
Pulsatile abdominal mass	History of untreated aneurysm

Therefore the pain or syncope becomes the focus of the work-up ("renal colic," "rule out cerebrovascular accident" or "rule out myocardial infarction"). It may not be until the terminal hypotensive episode that the diagnosis of RAAA is considered. An RAAA that is contained within the retroperitoneum may *not* cause hypotension or the typical presenting triad. The presence of peripheral pulses is *inconsequential* in the evaluation of RAAA. In the absence of hypotension, these patients may have *normal* femoral (or even distal) pulses, thereby providing an uninitiated examiner with a false sense of security.

Additional diagnostic tests. There are *no* laboratory tests diagnostic for RAAA, and many test results may be misleading. The patient with an RAAA may present with a mildly elevated white blood cell count and a normal hemoglobin level. Chemistry values are normal and an electrocardiogram may be confusing when it demonstrates signs of myocardial ischemia—

a result, rather than the cause, of the underlying disease process.

Judicious use of additional diagnostic examinations is indicated in a *stable* patient without the distinguishing characteristics of the diagnostic triad. A plain abdominal radiograph demonstrating a widened and calcified aorta or loss of the psoas muscle margins is suggestive of RAAA. However, the most accurate radiologic evaluation available for assessment of a possible RAAA remains the CT scan (Fig. 11-1). Most surgeons can easily interpret an abdominal CT scan, unlike ultrasound imaging, and technician-dependent factors

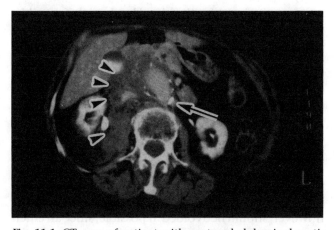

Fig. 11-1. CT scan of patient with ruptured abdominal aortic aneurysm. Rupture of abdominal aorta with dissection of blood through retroperitoneum *(arrowheads)*. The point of rupture *(arrow)* is most often posterolaterally on the left side of the aorta.

are limited. In addition, should the diagnosis of RAAA be incorrect, a CT scan may elucidate findings pertinent to the correct diagnosis. Percutaneous angiography is mentioned only to be condemned in the evaluation for *ruptured* AAA, since it is time-consuming and often will *not* identify an RAAA.

TREATMENT

Preoperative management and preparation. An RAAA requires operative treatment. Attempts at hemodynamic stabilization are contraindicated, since they unnecessarily delay transport of the patient to the operating room, thereby decreasing the patient's already low chance for survival. Peripheral intravenous access, a specimen for the blood bank, and, if possible, baseline hematologic and chemistry values and an electrocardiogram are all that should be obtained *en route* to the operating room. Central lines, chest radiographs, attempts at treating cardiac dysrhythmias (short of ventricular fibrillation) have no place in the emergency department management of these patients. A patient who is profoundly hypotensive on arrival at the hospital and whose response to fluid administration is minimal may undergo emergency thoracotomy to obtain proximal aortic control. This approach, however, should be avoided, if possible, since an emergency room thoracotomy is fraught with problems and is usually futile—even when performed by trained surgeons.

An integral part of the early management is alerting the operating room personnel. The nursing staff must move expeditiously to ready an operating room with appropriate instruments for both celiotomy *and* thoracotomy. Several circulating nurses are required to initiate the procedure, because tremendous demands are placed on them by both the surgeons and the anesthesiologists. Ideally, two anesthesiologists should be present to begin the procedure. A "cell saver" should be available to collect and reuse autogenous blood. The blood bank should be forewarned of the potential need for large quantities of blood products (red cells, fresh frozen plasma, cryoprecipitate, and platelets). The ambient temperature in the operating room must be raised to minimize heat loss (an important cause of fatal coagulopathies) during the operative procedure.

Preoperative preparation of the patient, including placement of a Foley catheter, insertion of hemodynamic monitoring equipment, skin preparation, draping with surgical sheets, and tracheal intubation should all be performed *before* anesthesia is induced. The patient must be forewarned of all the activity and should be constantly reassured that the actual surgery will not commence until he or she is fully anesthetized. Delaying the administration of anesthetic agents until the surgeon is ready to make the skin incision and obtain proximal control of the aorta is necessary, since it is common for the patient's blood pressure to drop precipitously when anesthesia is induced. This is caused by the loss of sympathetic tone that has, to this point, allowed for compensation of the large blood loss from the intravascular space.

Operation. After all necessary preparations have been made, the patient is anesthetized and exploration is begun through a long midline incision. The supraceliac approach to the aorta is a rapid and simple method of gaining aortic control. Distal aortic or iliac control is obtained with minimal dissection to avoid venous injury. Most vascular surgeons recommend moving the proximal clamp distal to the renal arteries before beginning the repair of an infrarenal aneurysm.

The choice of graft material is based on personal preference, but woven or coated grafts should be used to minimize bleeding in the face of coagulopathies. Expedience is mandatory when operating for RAAA but should not be achieved at the cost of deliberate and careful surgical technique.

Postoperative management. Postoperative management of these patients is complicated by the sequelae of preoperative and intraoperative episodes of prolonged hypotension. The immediate postoperative period generally requires aggressive maintenance of the circulating blood volume and correction of hypothermia and the induced coagulopathy. Postoperative management of fluid and electrolyte balance is complicated by the large amounts of fluids administered during the operation. The frequently concomitant presence of coronary artery disease mandates the use of a pulmonary artery catheter in all patients.

Renal failure is a frequent postoperative complication, and institution of dialysis must be considered *early* in the postoperative period to achieve maximal benefit. Pulmonary dysfunction resulting from fluid extravasation, respiratory distress syndrome, congestive heart failure, and underlying pulmonary disease necessitates aggressive pulmonary toilet. Other early postoperative complications include lower extremity ischemia, ischemic colitis, and bleeding. Management of the patient with an RAAA only *begins* with early recognition; the patient's *survival* depends on many factors, in addition to excellent intraoperative and postoperative care. The depth and duration of the hypotension are important factors; patients older than 80 years of age with impaired renal function or profound hypotension do not usually survive.

Vascular Trauma

The spectrum of vascular trauma ranges from simple laceration of a major artery or vein to the catastrophic disruption of the aorta with exsanguination. Evaluating a patient for vascular injury requires ascertaining the mechanism of injury, the elapsed time since the injury, and fully recognizing the extent of associated injuries. The patient's general condition should be continuously monitored, because the life of the patient must *never* be jeopardized in an effort to save a limb. The initial goal, hemostasis, may be achieved with direct pressure or angiographic embolization or it may necessitate more drastic measures, such as aortic cross-clamping. Once the hemorrhage is controlled, appropriate evaluation, followed by repair of the damaged vessels, can take place.

TRAUMA TO THE EXTREMITY

History. *Every* injured extremity must be evaluated for the presence of vascular injury. The history may raise the suspicion of vascular injuries, since certain mechanisms are associated with specific injuries (for example, posterior dislocations of the knee and popliteal artery thrombosis). Crush injuries to the extremity often involve arterial venous and nerve damage in addition to massive soft tissue destruction. Stab wounds are generally less devastating than gunshot wounds, which produce a blast effect (blunt trauma), compounding the penetrating bullet injury.

Physical examination. An accurate and thorough pulse examination, a detailed neurologic examination, and an assessment of bone, muscle, and soft tissue damage are essential. The decision to use additional diagnostic tests depends on the patient's history and the findings of the physical examination and the general condition of the patient. Exsanguinating hemorrhage requires direct pressure and immediate operative exploration; however, management of less obvious injuries is more controversial, with opinions ranging from mandatory exploration to selective use of arteriography or duplex scanning. Arteriography remains the gold standard for the nonoperative evaluation of arterial injury. The decision to proceed with arteriography is based on the presence of "soft" and "hard" signs of arterial injury (Table 11-2). If vascular injury is suspected, arteriography *should* be performed in a stable patient who does not require other operative intervention. Recently duplex ultrasonography has been advocated as a more sensitive and noninvasive modality for evaluating vascular injury. Although intimal flaps and subintimal hematomas have reportedly been managed nonoperatively, patients with these pathologic entities are best treated operatively unless the capacity exists to follow them closely with serial duplex scans. A limb that has been ischemic for more than 4 to 5 hours (6 hours is generally considered to be at the upper limit of "allowable ischemia time") requires immediate operative intervention, since the additional delay while obtaining an angiogram may jeopardize the viability of the extremity.

Table 11-2. Signs of Extremity Arterial Injury

"Hard" Signs	"Soft" Signs
Pulse deficit distal to injury	Proximity of missile or knife to major artery
Ischemia distal to injury	Adjacent nerve injury
Audible bruit	Unexplained hemorrhagic shock
Visible arterial bleeding	Significant swelling (out of proportion to injury)
Expanding or pulsatile hematoma	Moderate-sized, stable hematoma

The coexistence of a neurologic, orthopedic, or massive soft tissue injury in the presence of an arterial injury significantly decreases the chances for a successful functional outcome. Reperfusion must be established *before* repairing bony injuries—either by definitive repair or a temporary shunt. In performing the arterial repair, the surgeon must take into account the final adjusted length of the long bone after it is fixed by internal or external hardware, and the anastomosis *must be reinspected* following the orthopedic procedure.

TRAUMA TO THE GREAT VESSELS. Traumatic injuries to the aorta or subclavian or innominate arteries are usually fatal—most of these patients exsanguinate be-

---

Radiologic Signs Suggestive of Aortic or Brachiocephalic Arterial Rupture

Widened superior mediastinum
Loss of sharpness of aortic arch
Deviation of nasogastric tube to right
Downward displacement of left mainstem bronchus
Deviation of trachea to right
Apical cap sign
Enlarged or abnormal aortic contour
Left hemothorax

Modified from Perry MO. Arterial injuries: General principles of management. In Rutherford RB, ed. Vascular Surgery, 3rd ed. Philadelphia: WB Saunders, 1989, p 590.

fore they reach the hospital. A rupture of the thoracic aorta or innominate artery may *not* be immediately fatal, and patients who arrive in the hospital alive may have their diagnosis suspected on the basis of the initial chest radiograph (see the box on p. 206 and Fig. 11-2). Injury to the subclavian or innominate arteries

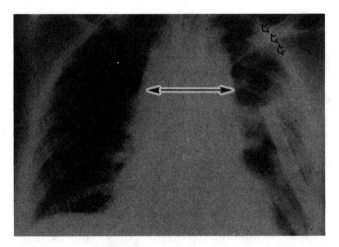

Fig. 11-2. Chest radiograph demonstrating typical findings of disruption of the aorta of great vessels. Pleural capping is seen at the superior aspect of the left lung fields *(open arrows)* and a widened mediastinum *(arrow)* is noted with loss of the aortic knob. The endotracheal tube has been displaced to the right and a left hemothorax has been partially treated via a tube thoracostomy. (From Oreskovich MR, Carrico CJ. Trauma: Management of the acutely injured patient. In Sabiston DC, Jr, ed. Textbook of Surgery, 13th ed. Philadelphia: WB Saunders, 1986, p 306.)

often presents as massive hemothorax, with the exact location of the injury undiagnosed before thoracotomy is performed. If a diagnosis of injury to the innominate or right subclavian artery or aortic arch is made preoperatively, surgical exploration is performed via a median sternotomy; however, the left subclavian artery is best approached through a left thoracotomy for control of hemorrhage and repair of the injured vessel.

Injury to the carotid artery may present as an expanding neck hematoma, profuse bleeding, or a neurologic deficit. The use of arteriography is encouraged in the nonoperative management of penetrating neck trauma, as are bronchoscopy and esophagoscopy or contrast esophagography. Indications for carotid arterial repair include the presence of an expanding hematoma or persistent bleeding from the neck. An injury to the carotid artery in the *absence* of a comatose state is also an indication for operative repair. A comatose patient with a nonbleeding carotid artery injury should *not* undergo repair, since the acutely ischemic cortex may undergo hemorrhagic degeneration if perfusion is reestablished. Should the need for hemostasis mandate operative exploration, the carotid artery should be ligated rather than repaired operatively. The noncomatose patient with a carotid arterial injury should undergo primary repair or placement of an interposition graft, if necessary. Injuries to the carotid artery close to the skull base require more complex operative repair, including subluxation of the mandible, external to internal carotid artery bypass, or insertion of shunts or occluding material, with ligation of the proximal internal carotid artery to control the hemorrhage.

PELVIC FRACTURES AND RETROPERITONEAL HEMORRHAGE. Pelvic fractures are notorious for their associated blood loss. This often massive hemorrhage is caused by disruption of the pelvic and presacral plexus of veins as a result of the shifting bony structures of the pelvis. If appropriate fluid and blood replacement is given, quite often the bleeding will stop. However, should hemorrhage persist, the mainstay of therapy in these patients is to stabilize the pelvic fracture with external fixation. If blood loss continues *after* pelvic stabilization, it is usually from an arterial source. These situations are best treated by selective arteriographic embolization of the bleeding vessels.

Although embolization is the preferred treatment, a trauma surgeon often operates on a patient with a severe pelvic fracture for *another* intra-abdominal injury. When a retroperitoneal hematoma is encountered in this situation, it *must not be entered*. Although bilateral internal iliac artery ligation has been advocated, the results are generally unsatisfactory. In a patient with severe pelvic fractures and significant bleeding from the pelvic and presacral plexus, these vessels should be tamponaded with laparotomy pads while the other intraperitoneal injuries are repaired. If pelvic hemorrhage is present at the conclusion of the operation, the celiotomy incision should be closed and the patient transported to the angiography suite for an attempt at embolization. Direct suture repair of these injuries is often not possible.

VENOUS TRAUMA. Most venous injuries may be treated safely by ligating the injured vein. Attempts at repair should be performed *only* in patients who are otherwise stable and have no indication for other operative intervention. Injuries to the vena cava and iliac veins may be repaired primarily or, rarely, with the use of an interposition prosthetic graft. The deep venous system of the lower extremities is best repaired primarily or by using a saphenous vein graft from the contralateral leg, if available. Ligation is generally well tolerated; however, the sequelae must be recognized and actions taken to counter their effects in the early postoperative period. Lower extremity edema, which impedes wound healing, is caused by the decreased venous outflow and compounded by the massive fluid load routinely given trauma victims in the perioperative period. Leg elevation and sequential compression devices aid in countering the effects of edema; however, the long-term complications of venous stasis including ulceration, chronic edema, and recurrent infections may require constant attention.

COMPARTMENT SYNDROME. Although compartment syndrome may occur in any fascia-contained compartment of the body, it is most commonly encountered in the leg. The syndrome develops when the interstitial pressure within a compartment exceeds that of the venous pressure within that space. The result is progressive nerve and muscle ischemia that, if untreated, results in myonecrosis and neurologic damage.

Diagnosis. The diagnosis is primarily a clinical one, and the index of suspicion must be high with *any* injury to the extremity. The patient may be asymptomatic or may have a decrease or loss of sensation in the first dorsal web space of the foot, pain in the calf on dorsiflexion of the ankle joint, tenderness of the calf muscles, or, finally, loss of distal pulses. Compartmental pressures can be measured using either an elaborate manometry system or a simple intravenous catheter and three-way stopcock attached to a sphygmomanometer. Doppler ultrasound has been used to aid in the diagnosis of compartment syndrome, since compression-augmented venous flow will cease when the tissue pressure within a compartment exceeds that of the venous pressure.

Treatment. Once the diagnosis has been made, *urgent* fasciotomy is indicated. The liberal use of fasciotomies (even prophylactically) in trauma is advocated, since it is not uncommon for myonecrosis to occur in the presence of "normal" compartment pressures. Should the muscles within the compartments not have the typical dusky colored, bulging appearance seen in compartment syndrome, the wounds may be closed primarily in several days.

The lower leg has four separate compartments (Fig. 11-3) that must *all* be decompressed during the fasciotomy procedure. The procedure is performed through two separate incisions—anterolateral and posteromedial—and some surgeons advocate the need for a fibulectomy. Although the anterior compartment is the one at greatest risk, *all four* compartments must be adequately decompressed before terminating the procedure.

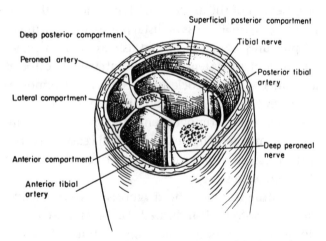

Fig. 11-3. The four anatomic compartments of the lower leg are identified with their neurovascular structures. (From Perry MO. Compartment syndromes and reperfusion injury. Surg Clin North Am 68:859, 1988.)

Diabetic Foot Infections

Including the management of diabetic foot infections in a section dedicated to vascular emergencies underscores the malignant nature of this disease. The outcome of a diabetic patient with a foot infection depends on immediate recognition, rapid correction of metabolic derangements, and aggressive, timely surgical intervention. The consequences of mismanagement in these cases are loss of a limb, at the least, and possibly loss of life.

ETIOLOGIC FACTORS. The patient with diabetes mellitus is at significantly high risk for developing an infection of the lower extremity. The microcirculation in these patients (vessels distal to the larger named arteries) is frequently diseased, thus producing a relatively ischemic environment for bacteria to proliferate. The suppressed state of the diabetic's immune system is another factor that predisposes the patient to infection. Diabetic neuropathy results in an insensate foot that is prone to unnoticed trauma, retention of foreign bodies for prolonged periods, and an inability to recognize the pain of infection when it is present within the deep, closed spaces of the foot.

DIAGNOSIS. The importance of immediate diagnosis and recognizing that a diabetic foot infection is an emergency cannot be overemphasized. Most patients with diabetes mellitus who develop an infection of their foot present with obvious signs and symptoms of infection, including fever, discoloration (erythema or gangrene), edema, a malodorous discharge, and possibly, pain.

However, pain and tenderness may *not* be present if the diabetic neuropathy is severe. When the infection is contained within the deep spaces of the foot by the plantar fascia, overt signs of infection may be absent. Mild tenderness or erythema along the dorsal aspect of the foot represents the "tip of the iceberg" and must raise the examiner's suspicion, prompting a more extensive evaluation. A small amount of purulent discharge, which may look relatively benign, may signify an extensive deep plantar abscess. Therefore *any patient with diabetes mellitus who presents with fever must be closely examined for infection of the lower extremity.* Some advanced infections in diabetic patients are associated with gas formation and crepitus. This rarely signifies gas gangrene or clostridial sepsis.

If a closed-space foot infection *is* suspected, other diagnostic maneuvers may be performed. Although recent reports suggest a role for magnetic resonance imaging in identifying occult abscesses in the diabetic foot, it is an expensive procedure and the equipment is not universally available. Needle aspiration with an 18-gauge needle and sterile technique will often locate the purulent material of an abscess cavity. Aspirated material should be cultured (aerobically and anaerobically) and Gram stained to identify the predominant organism or organisms. If no abscess cavity is identified and no necrotic or gangrenous tissue is present but a deep foot infection is still suspected, operative exploration is indicated.

MANAGEMENT

Medical. Management of diabetic foot infections is straightforward: stabilize the patient, drain the infection, and administer antibiotics. Once the infection has been recognized, a sense of urgency *must* develop. Diabetic ketoacidosis may occur as a result of the evolving septic process within the foot. Routine blood chemistry values, arterial blood gas evaluations, and peripheral blood cultures should be obtained before antibiotics are administered. Catheterization of the urinary bladder may be necessary for fluid management, and placement of a pulmonary artery or central venous catheter may be required in a patient with associated severe congestive failure or unstable angina.

Although it is preferable to have the medical problems stabilized before surgical drainage is undertaken, this is often not possible, since the infection may be responsible for the patient's condition. Should the patient be too ill to transport, a bedside drainage procedure—although usually inadequate—performed with local or regional anesthesia may reverse a rapidly deteriorating course. This may allow time for further management before performing the complete operative excision and drainage.

Operative. Operative drainage is the cornerstone of treatment for diabetic foot infections. The drainage procedure should be immediate and aggressive, leaving *no* infected or necrotic tissue behind (excision and drainage). Amputations of digits, transmetatarsal amputations, or partial leg amputations are usually required and should be performed *without hesitation*— because an aggressive approach will allow the patient to retain the remainder of the limb and will save his life. Incomplete drainage and debridement allow further spread of the infection, with more tissue loss than if the original amputation and excision of necrotic tissue had been satisfactorily performed. The wounds should generally be left open at initial operation, with delayed primary closure or skin grafting at a later date.

Antibiotics. Published reports have *not* demonstrated any antibiotic to be superior, since most diabetic foot infections are caused by mixed organisms including *Staphylococcus, Streptococcus, Enterobacter,* and *Bacteroides* species. Therefore the antibiotics must be chosen with consideration given to spectrum, toxicity, and cost. Although monotherapy is attractive for its ease of administration, the cost is often prohibitive. Two- and three-drug regimens offer a broad spectrum of coverage, but they require larger volumes of fluid administration. Use of aminoglycosides should be avoided, since most patients with diabetes mellitus have some degree of preexisting renal insufficiency. Antibiotics should be administered *immediately* after the blood cultures are obtained and be continued until the wound has no obvious signs of infection.

Careful postoperative care includes correction of metabolic derangements and aggressive wound care. Appropriate and frequent dressing changes, hydrotherapy, physical therapy, and bedside debridements are of utmost importance to preserve the maximum length and function of the affected limb.

Iatrogenic Injuries

This section focuses on iatrogenic injuries that occur as the result of arterial punctures for diagnostic or therapeutic interventional procedures. Therapeutic procedures such as angioplasty necessitate frequent catheter changes, and the caliber of the sheaths and catheters is generally larger than those used for diagnostic purposes. The complications of arterial catheterization can be divided into two categories: thrombotic and, the more common, hemorrhagic.

THROMBOTIC COMPLICATIONS

Etiologic factors. Atherosclerotic plaques, if dislodged from the site of arterial puncture, can produce thrombosis, distal embolization, and ischemia. Despite appropriate anticoagulation, an intraluminal clot may form on the catheter sheath, thereby precipitating thrombus formation, or it may be carried distally by arterial flow as a thromboembolus.

Diagnosis

History and physical examination. Pain in the catheterized extremity mandates a thorough evaluation by an experienced examiner. Attributing the pain to the puncture itself is dangerous and fraught with the complications of prolonged extremity ischemia—namely limb loss. Signs and symptoms of ischemia include the following:

- Pain
- Mottling of the skin
- Cyanosis or marked difference in cutaneous temperature between limbs

Examination may reveal the following:

- Hypersensitivity to palpation
- Pain on flexion of ischemic muscle groups (e.g., calf pain on ankle dorsiflexion)
- Hypesthesia

An accurate pulse examination is the essential first step in evaluation. Unfortunately, there is often an inadequate or unreliable pulse examination documented in the precatheterization medical record. Pulse evaluation of the contralateral extremity is helpful, because the presence of occlusive disease *tends* to be symmetric. A history of claudication or the results of previous noninvasive or angiographic evaluations are also useful in this regard. Although an accurate pulse examination often provides the necessary information to assist in determining the therapeutic approach, further diagnostic examinations may be required.

Additional diagnostic tests. Ankle-brachial indices are easy to perform and may yield additional information. A Doppler flow evaluation is often misinterpreted and will provide an uninitiated examiner with a false sense of security. The presence of an audible Doppler signal does *not* ensure flow that is adequate for limb viability. Pulse volume recordings and arteriography are examinations that allow determination of the adequacy of the blood supply; however, the clinical picture, coupled with an accurate pulse examination, may be all that is required to develop an appropriate therapeutic plan.

Treatment. Rapid restoration of adequate blood flow is essential to prevent limb loss and the consequences of reperfusion injury. Preoperative angiography is of great value in determining the operative plan. In the absence of this study, however, emphasis must be placed on the pulse examination. The presence of a strong femoral pulse in the injured extremity indicates an occlusion distal to the inguinal ligament.

Exploration of the femoral artery, using local anesthesia, allows repair of the injured vessel at the catheterization site and passage of embolectomy catheters for removal of thromboembolic material. If an angiogram has not been obtained preoperatively, one may be obtained in the operating room through the proximal arteriotomy.

Exposure of the below-knee popliteal artery may be preferable, since embolectomy catheters can be passed proximally into the superficial and common femoral arteries as well as distally into the infrapopliteal trifurcation vessels. Thromboembolectomy may be inadequate for restoring circulation to the foot. An arterial bypass may be required, emphasizing the necessity of adequately preparing the patient and the operative field in advance for a major procedure.

HEMORRHAGIC COMPLICATIONS. Complications of hemostasis are more common in arterial catheterization than are thrombotic complications. These may manifest as hypovolemic shock, hematoma or pseudoaneurysm formation, arteriovenous fistulas or dissection of the arterial wall.

Etiologic factors. Although catheter technology has progressed since the first coronary angioplasty was performed, an 8 or 9 Fr sheath is still required for most interventional cardiac procedures. The common practice of postangioplasty heparinization has increased the rate of hemorrhagic complications. Inadvertent passage of the catheter through the posterior wall of the artery allows hemorrhage into the thigh, since direct pressure might not produce adequate hemostasis. Perforation of the iliac or proximal femoral artery can cause bleeding into the retroperitoneal space, thereby producing hypovolemic shock.

The development of a pseudoaneurysm at the site of an arterial puncture results from inadequate compression of the puncture site after removal of the catheter sheath. Direct pressure must be maintained long enough to ensure hemostasis—especially in a patient who has undergone a full course of anticoagulation therapy. The formation of an arteriovenous fistula, resulting from inadvertent puncture of the femoral vein, has been reported more frequently when simultaneous femoral artery and femoral vein catheterizations are performed in the same side of the groin for left- and right-sided heart catheterization, respectively.

Diagnosis

Hypovolemia. Hypotension following catheterization is often attributed to cardiac failure, since the primary focus of the patient's care has been the cardiac disease. Instituting therapy for cardiogenic shock in the patient with excessive blood loss is inappropriate and possibly fatal. Serial hematocrit levels should be routinely checked following catheterization procedures, and a significant drop in either the hematocrit or the systolic blood pressure must be investigated with a CT scan of the retroperitoneum and possibly the thigh.

Pseudoaneurysm versus hematoma. Bleeding into the thigh is common, as evidenced by the frequency of hematoma formation at arterial puncture sites. Distinguishing a groin hematoma from a pseudoaneurysm (Fig. 11-4) is often difficult on the basis of physical findings; pain and the size of the mass are *not* useful distinguishing characteristics. The presence of pulsations within the mass may not differentiate the two either, since the femoral arterial pulse may often be palpated through a hematoma (Table 11-3). A bruit, more common in a pseudoaneurysm, may be auscultated when a hematoma is impinging on the arterial flow. Although angiography has been the standard procedure for demonstrating the presence of a pseudoaneurysm, duplex ultrasonography (Fig. 11-5) may also distinguish a pseudoaneurysm from a hematoma. The duplex scan is not only diagnostic but also has recently been reported to be a useful therapeutic modality in treating catheter-related pseudoaneurysms.

Arteriovenous fistulas. Arteriovenous fistulas are diagnosed on physical examination in the presence of a palpable thrill and a *continuous* bruit over the puncture site. Rarely are these fistulas large enough to cause congestive heart failure by acutely increasing the preload of the right heart. Angiography will document

Table 11-3. Differentiating Hematoma From Pseudoaneurysm

Parameter	Hematoma	Pseudoaneurysm
Pain	Present	Present
Size	Variable	Variable
Pulsatile	Occasionally	Usually (if not thrombosed)
Bruit	Possible	Present
Angiogram	Normal	Abnormal
Duplex scan	Normal (may see hematoma)	Abnormal (extra-anatomic flow seen)

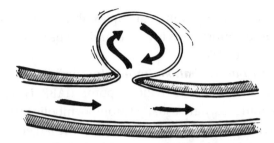

Fig. 11-4. Schematic representation of a pseudoaneurysm. Note the disruption of the intimal continuity with persistent flow in the vessel. The flow extrinsic to the main vessel is contained within a fibrous capsule.

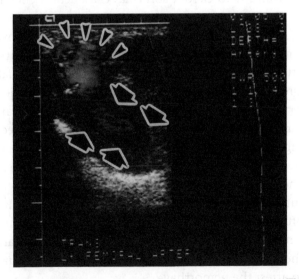

Fig. 11-5. Duplex ultrasound of a femoral pseudoaneurysm. The intimal continuity *(broad arrows)* has been disrupted and flow within the pseudoaneurysm *(arrowheads)* is demonstrated.

these communications, but duplex ultrasonography is easier to perform, less invasive, and can be done at the patient's bedside.

Intra-aortic balloon pump. Injuries encountered when an intra-aortic balloon pump (IABP) is placed percutaneously are usually thromboembolic but may be hemorrhagic, in part as a result of the larger size of the catheter sheath required for their introduction. Iliac or femoral artery thrombosis is readily diagnosed on physical examination by the absence of a femoral pulse. Intimal flaps, arterial wall dissection, and emboli from an atherosclerotic aorta may cause acute ischemia.

Treatment

Hypovolemia. The definitive treatment for hypovolemic hemorrhagic shock is operative repair of the artery. Halting heparin therapy, restoring an adequate circulating blood volume, and transporting the patient to the operating room constitute appropriate therapy for the patient with documented retroperitoneal bleeding that is causing hemodynamic instability. Operative repair may be performed under local anesthesia and, quite often, routine exposure of the artery with suture repair of an arterial wall defect will suffice. It is often desirable, however, to avoid operating on these patients. Frequently in these cases, cessation of heparin therapy with blood replacement may prove adequate to arrest the hemorrhage.

Pseudoaneurysm. The most severe complication of an ***arterial pseudoaneurysm*** (PA) is rupture. Advocates of conservative therapy for small PAs (less than 2 cm) have documented the frequency with which PAs resolve with conservative management. Recent reports suggest that the experienced duplex ultrasonographer can locate and compress the exact point of arterial disruption (while maintaining distal arterial flow), effecting obliteration of the PA over several hours. However, this technique requires time and experienced personnel and must at this time be considered preliminary. Surgical repair of a PA involves identification and suture repair of the arterial wall defect. Opinions differ as to the appropriate method of gaining control of the artery being repaired—either clamping the vessel proximal and distal to the PA sac or obtaining intrasaccular control. Regardless of the method used, careful vascular technique must be used in closing the defect to avoid narrowing of the artery at the site of injury.

Infected pseudoaneurysms may present months after the catheterization procedure. This entity requires a different operative approach—ligation and exclusion of the PA with an arterial bypass graft that is tunneled outside the area of infection.

Arteriovenous fistulas. Arteriovenous fistulas (AVF) occur when there is a direct communication between an artery and a vein. This is usually the result of a needle puncturing the back wall of an artery and the anterior wall of the vein, thereby establishing this anomalous communication. Surgical repair of an AVF requires suture ligation of the fistula from *within* the arterial lumen. These procedures can sometimes be performed using local anesthesia. Early repair of an AVF minimizes the risk of late complications such as congestive failure, deep venous thrombosis, or arterial embolization.

Intra-aortic balloon pump. IABP-induced injuries are often noted early in their course. The complications encountered in these patients are similar to those described earlier. However, these patients are generally sicker than are cardiac catheterization patients, hence the reason for their requiring the IABP. Treatment is dictated by the severity of their presenting problem—either hemorrhagic or thrombotic—with special attention given to their tenuous medical condition.

BIBLIOGRAPHY
Ruptured Abdominal Aortic Aneurysms

Mannick JA, Whittemore AD. Management of ruptured or symptomatic abdominal aortic aneurysms. Surg Clin North Am 68:377-384, 1988.

Rutherford RB, McCroskey BL. Ruptured abdominal aortic aneurysms: Special considerations. Surg Clin North Am 69:859-868, 1989.

Veith FJ, Gupta S, Daly V. Technique for occluding the supraceliac aorta through the abdomen. Surg Gynecol Obstet 151:426-428, 1980.

Veith FJ, Gupta SK, Wengerter KW. Emergency abdominal aortic aneurysm surgery and supraceliac aortic control. In Greenhalgh RM, Mannick JA, eds. The Cause and Management of Aneurysms. London: WB Saunders Ltd, 1990, pp 387-400.

Vascular Trauma

Feliciano DV, Hershkowitz K, O'Gorman RB, Cruse PA, Brandt ML, Burch JM, Mattox KL. Management of vascular injuries in the lower extremities. J Trauma 28:319-328, 1988.

Liekwig WG, Greenfield LJ. Management of penetrating carotid arterial injury. Ann Surg 188:587-592, 1978.

McCroskey BL, Moore EE, Rutherford RB, eds. Vascular Trauma. Surg Clin North Am 68:683-890, 1988.

Perry MO. Complications of missed arterial injuries. J Vasc Surg 17:399-407, 1993.

Perry MO, Snyder WH, Thal ER. Carotid artery injuries caused by blunt trauma. Ann Surg 192:74-77, 1980.

Diabetic Foot Infections

Towne JB. Management of foot lesions in the diabetic patient. In Rutherford RB, ed. Vascular Surgery, 3rd ed. Philadelphia: WB Saunders, 1989, pp 783-791.

Iatrogenic Injuries

Feld R, Patton GM, Carabasi A, Alexander A, Merton D, Needleman L. Treatment of iatrogenic femoral artery injuries with ultrasound-guided compression. J Vasc Surg 16:832-840, 1992.

Kresowik TF, Khoury MD, Miller BV, Winniford MD, Shamma AR, Sharp WJ, Blecha MB, Corson JD. A prospective study of the incidence and natural history of femoral vascular complications after percutaneous transluminal coronary angioplasty. J Vasc Surg 13:328-335, 1991.

Oweida SW, Roubin GS, Smith RB III, Salam AA. Postcatheterization vascular complications associated with percutaneous transluminal coronary angioplasty. J Vasc Surg 12:310-315, 1990.

12
Vascular Disease of the Upper Extremity

Hannah L. Brooks

Thoracic Outlet Syndrome

Thoracic outlet syndrome (TOS) is characterized by neurologic, venous, and arterial abnormalities resulting from compression of the subclavian vessels or brachial plexus as they exit the thorax. This may be produced by bony or soft tissue anomalies of the scalene triangle (Figs. 12-1 and 12-2). TOS is usually seen in women (3:1) 20 to 40 years of age. The symptomatology depends on the structures being compressed (nerve, vein, or artery) (Fig. 12-3).

NEUROLOGIC. Compression of the brachial plexus is responsible for 95% of the cases of TOS. The most common cause of neurologic compression is soft tissue abnormalities. Pain and paresthesias, usually in the *ulnar* nerve distribution, are the most common presenting complaints. Motor weakness occurs in 10% of patients with neurologic TOS. The differential diagnosis of upper extremity neurologic abnormalities includes TOS, cervical radiculopathy, and carpal tunnel syndrome. Cervical radiculopathy usually occurs in a

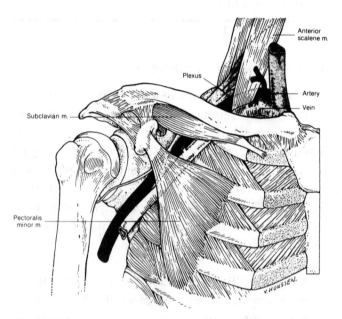

Fig. 12-1. The anterior scalene muscle divides the thoracic outlet into an anterior compartment containing the subclavian vein and a posterior compartment, the scalene triangle, containing subclavian artery and brachial plexus. (From Heberer G, van Donegen RJAM. Vascular Surgery. Berlin: Springer-Verlag, 1988, p 554.)

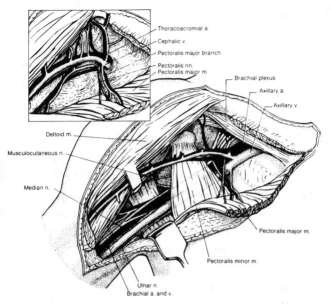

Fig. 12-2. Anatomy of the thoracic outlet. (From Heberer G, van Donegen RJAM. Vascular Surgery. Berlin: Springer-Verlag, 1988, p 20.)

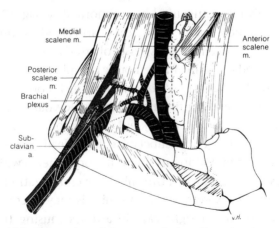

Fig. 12-3. Orientation of neurovascular bundle and scalene muscles. (From Heberer G, van Donegen RJAM. Vascular Surgery. Berlin: Springer-Verlag, 1988, p 554.)

radial nerve distribution and carpal tunnel syndrome in a *medial* nerve distribution, whereas TOS occurs in the C8 to T1 *ulnar* nerve distribution.

VENOUS. Venous compression occurs in 4% of patients with TOS. It is characterized by edema, cyanosis and sensations of heaviness or tingling in the affected upper extremity. The symptoms may begin after exercise (effort thrombosis). The resultant subclavian vein thrombosis may produce engorged venous collaterals or a palpable cord in the arm.

ARTERIAL. Arterial compression occurs in 1% of patients with TOS. It is more common on the right side due to the higher takeoff of the right subclavian artery from the innominate artery and is caused almost exclusively by a congenital *bony* abnormality (Fig. 12-4). This produces coldness, weakness, and claudication of the upper extremity. Most cases of arterial TOS are not diagnosed until thromboembolic complications have occurred. Patients may note nonhealing lesions or pallor in the hands or fingers. Unilateral Raynaud's phenomenon, although infrequent, can also occur. Chronic compression of the subclavian artery leads to stenosis or poststenotic aneurysm formation, either of which can serve as a nidus for thrombosis or embolization. In rare instances, retrograde thrombosis may affect the vertebral and/or right carotid arteries causing transient ischemic attacks or stroke.

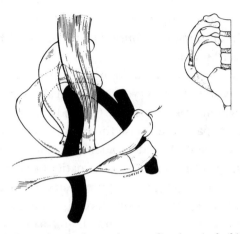

Fig. 12-4. Example of a bony abnormality (cervical rib) and its associated vascular compression. (From Heberer G, van Donegen RJAM. Vascular Surgery. Berlin: Springer-Verlag, 1988, p 553.)

PHYSICAL EXAMINATION. Initial inspection of the patient presenting with TOS may reveal bony asymmetry, muscular atrophy, venous engorgement, pallor of the hand or arm, focal ischemia, or a gangrenous lesion (blue finger syndrome).

The pulse in the affected arm may be absent or diminished, and a blood pressure differential of at least 20 mm Hg between the upper extremities may exist. A subclavian artery bruit, suggestive of stenosis, can be auscultated. Bony abnormalities or a pulsatile supraclavicular mass may be palpable. Neurologic testing may demonstrate paresthesia, hypesthesia, or anesthesia in an ulnar distribution or weakness of the interosseous muscles.

A number of provocative maneuvers may be used to elicit symptoms of TOS during physical examination. The ***elevated arm stress test*** (EAST) is performed by having the patient exercise the hands with elbows at 90 degrees and shoulders abducted and externally rotated. This can reproduce the patient's symptoms. ***Adson's test,*** although of disputed value, is performed by having the patient inspire forcibly, rotate the head toward the side being examined, and forcibly place the shoulders back in the military position while the examiner monitors the quality of the radial pulse.

DIAGNOSIS. When TOS is suspected, cervical spine and chest radiographs should be obtained. Bony abnormalities (cervical rib, bifid first rib) or soft tissue abnormalities (superior mediastinal masses) are often evident on plain radiographs.

Duplex scanning of the subclavian artery may identify poststenotic dilatation (aneurysm), mural thrombus or arterial occlusion. Pulse volume recordings are an objective method to assess arterial circulation in the extremity.

Although electromyelograms are rarely employed, they may aid in localizing a nerve compression across or *distal* to the thoracic outlet.

Angiography is mandatory in patients exhibiting signs of upper extremity arterial or venous thromboembolism. It may also be indicated in patients with a documented bony abnormality of the thoracic outlet, so that surgical correction may be undertaken before the onset of ischemic complications.

Stenosis of the subclavian artery at the thoracic outlet with a poststenotic dilatation can be demonstrated angiographically. When a venous cause of TOS is suspected, duplex examination or venography should be performed.

TREATMENT. The initial treatment for TOS of a neurologic origin involves physical therapy and muscle relaxants. Surgery is indicated for those with unremitting, disabling symptoms. The best surgical results have been reported with anterior scalenectomy and first rib (or cervical rib) resection. This can be performed through a transaxillary (Fig. 12-5) or supraclavicular approach.

Patients with TOS caused by venous compression will often benefit from nonoperative management. Resolution of symptoms will occur in two thirds of patients undergoing a course of elevation and anticoagulation therapy. Patients whose symptoms do not remit within 2 to 3 days of conservative therapy may require more aggressive management. A decision to perform venous thrombectomy must be made early, before the intravascular clot has organized. In the last several years, thrombolytic therapy has been advocated in cases in which venous thrombosis has been present for less than 3 weeks. When successful, this should

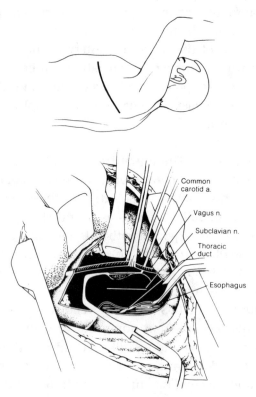

Fig. 12-5. Transaxillary approach to neurovascular and bony structures. (From Heberer G, van Donegen RJAM. Vascular Surgery. Berlin: Springer-Verlag, 1988, p 271.)

be followed by balloon dilatation of residual vein stenoses and first rib resection. Venous bypass is of questionable value and is reserved for those patients who fail conservative management and develop a severe postphlebitic syndrome.

Patients with arterial TOS generally present with acutely ischemic symptoms of the upper extremity. When poststenotic dilation of the subclavian artery occurs in conjunction with embolic events, *simple ligation of the aneurysm is contraindicated.* Embolectomy alone without correction of the underlying abnormality is also contraindicated.

Following arteriography, management of these patients is surgical. Although the transaxillary approach can be used (it allows for excision of a cervical or first rib), it may not offer adequate exposure of the subclavian artery. Using the supraclavicular approach (Figs. 12-6 and 12-7), bony resection may be accomplished along with arterial reconstruction as needed. Distal thromboembolectomies may also be required.

When poststenotic dilation of the subclavian artery is minimal, the treatment of arterial TOS remains controversial. Although some authors believe that these lesions regress after removal of the compressive structure alone, others advocate subclavian arteriotomy to inspect for intimal lesions or thrombi. The advent of angioscopy may obviate the need for long arteriotomies in these cases.

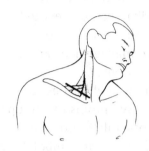

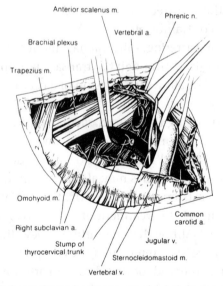

Anterior scalenus m.

Phrenic n.

Vertebral a.

Brachial plexus

Trapezius m.

Omohyoid m.

Common carotid a.

Right subclavian a.

Jugular v.

Stump of thyrocervical trunk

Sternocleidomastoid m.

Vertebral v.

Fig. 12-6. Supraclavicular exposure of subclavian artery aneurysm. (From Heberer G, van Donegen RJAM. Vascular Surgery. Berlin: Springer-Verlag, 1988, p 272.)

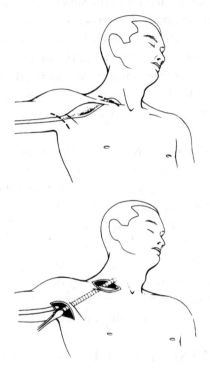

Fig. 12-7. Transclavicular exposure of thoracic outlet. (From Heberer G, van Donegen RJAM. Vascular Surgery. Berlin: Springer-Verlag, 1988, p 272.)

Cervical Rib

Complete cervical rib, fused or articulated to the first thoracic rib lateral to the subclavian artery, is the most common bony abnormality in patients with *arterial* complications of TOS. *Incomplete* cervical ribs, with a fibrous band attached to the first rib, are, when symptomatic, more commonly associated with *neurologic* TOS (Fig. 12-8). When present, cervical ribs are bilateral in approximately 75% of cases.

PHYSICAL EXAMINATION. Many of the signs of cervical rib have been outlined in the section on TOS. The cervical rib may be palpated, and, in the absence of subclavian artery thrombosis, a harsh bruit is usually present in the supraclavicular fossa.

DIAGNOSIS. The presence of a cervical rib is evident on radiographs. Arteriography is necessary in all cases, regardless of symptoms, to assess the degree of poststenotic dilation of the subclavian artery.

TREATMENT. Operation is indicated in those displaying upper extremity ischemia. Supraclavicular and transaxillary approaches have been recommended. The supraclavicular approach has been advocated by those who believe scalenectomy must be included at operation, and it allows inspection and treatment of the subclavian artery as well as excision of compressive bony structures.

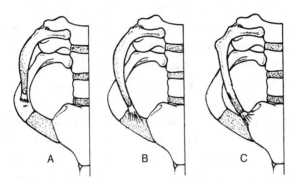

Fig. 12-8. A, Cervical rib with fibrous band. **B**, Incomplete cervical rib with cartilage. **C**, Complete cervical rib. (From Heberer G, van Donegen RJAM. Vascular Surgery. Berlin: Springer-Verlag, 1988, p 554.)

Subclavian Steal Syndrome

Subclavian steal syndrome (SSS) occurs when a stenosis or occlusion of the subclavian or innominate artery exists proximal to the vertebral artery. It is characterized by retrograde flow in the vertebral artery to the ipsilateral postocclusive subclavian artery.

PHYSICAL EXAMINATION. Decreased pulses are noted in the affected limb, as is a supraclavicular bruit. Symptoms are reproduced by exercising the arm on the same side of the lesion.

DIAGNOSIS. Symptoms of SSS can be related to either cerebral or brachial arterial insufficiency. Many patients report dizziness, vertigo, upper extremity claudication, paresis and paresthesias. The *left* subclavian is implicated twice as frequently as the right.

Diagnostic studies. Angiography, demonstrating subclavian stenosis with reversal of flow in the vertebral artery, is the standard method for diagnosing SSS. If the stenotic lesion is atherosclerotic in nature, a careful examination for a coexistent carotid lesion should be performed. Although many patients demonstrate an anatomic SSS on angiography, few will actually have symptoms. It is the symptomatic patient with a dominant vertebral artery on the side of the lesion that should be considered for operative repair.

TREATMENT. Intervention is indicated when SSS causes symptoms of vertebrobasilar insufficiency or disabling upper extremity claudication. Transluminal angioplasty may be considered for the treatment of short segmental stenoses of the subclavian artery.

Operative management of SSS is best accomplished by an extrathoracic approach. The carotid-subclavian bypass, using synthetic graft material, is performed through a supraclavicular approach (Fig. 12-9). Other options include an extra-anatomic subclavian-subclavian bypass (Fig. 12-10) or implantation of the subclavian into the common carotid artery (Fig 12-11). Po-

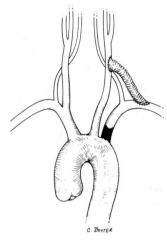

Fig. 12-9. Standard carotid-subclavian bypass. (From Greenhalgh R. Indications in Vascular Surgery. Philadelphia: WB Saunders, 1988, p 64.)

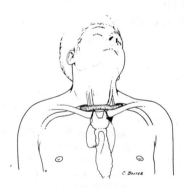

Fig. 12-10. Subclavian-subclavian bypass. (From Greenhalgh R. Indications in Vascular Surgery. Philadelphia: WB Saunders, 1988, p 65.)

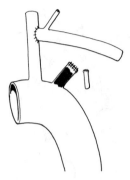

Fig. 12-11. Subclavian artery transposition. (From Greenhalgh R. Indications in Vascular Surgery. Philadelphia: WB Saunders, 1988, p 76.)

tential complications of these operations include thoracic duct and phrenic nerve injury. The advantages of these techniques, however, are that they correct retrograde flow in the vertebral artery.

BIBLIOGRAPHY

Barwegen MGMH, van Donegen RJAM. Compression syndromes. In Heberer G, van Donegen RJAM, eds. Vascular Surgery. Berlin: Springer-Verlag, 1988, pp 553-566.

Clagett GP. Upper extremity aneurysms. In Rutherford RB, ed. Vascular Surgery, 3rd ed. Philadelphia: WB Saunders, 1989, pp 957-969.

Denck H. Reconstructive operations in the area of the subclavian and axillary artery. In Greenhalgh R, ed. Indications in Vascular Surgery. Philadelphia: WB Saunders, 1988, pp 73-89.

Kieffer E, Ruotolo C. Arterial complications of thoracic outlet compression. In Rutherford RB, ed. Vascular Surgery, 3rd ed. Philadelphia: WB Saunders, 1989, pp 875-882.

Mannick J. Extrathoracic operations for lesions of the vessels arising from the aortic arch. In Greenhalgh R, ed. Indications in Vascular Surgery. Philadelphia: WB Saunders, 1988, pp 63-69.

Pilcher DB, Davis JH. Aorta and peripheral arteries. In Davis JH, ed. Clinical Surgery. St. Louis: CV Mosby Co, 1987, p 2157.

Roos DB. Thoracic Outlet Nerve Compression. In Rutherford RB, ed. Vascular Surgery, 3rd ed. Philadelphia: WB Saunders, 1989, pp. 858-875.

Rutherford RB, Piotrowski JJ. Axillary-subclavian vein thrombosis. In Rutherford RB, ed. Vascular Surgery, 3rd ed. Philadelphia: WB Saunders, 1989, pp 883-889.

Scher LA, Veith FJ, Haimovici H, Samson RH, Ascer E, Gupta SK, Sprayregen S. Staging of arterial complications of cervical rib: Guidelines for surgical management. Surgery 95:644-649, 1984.

13

Nonatherosclerotic Vascular Disease

Arthur T. Martella

Atherosclerosis accounts for the large majority of occlusive vascular disease. However, there is a group of disorders that must be considered in evaluating patients with ischemic disease, particularly those with upper extremity symptoms and an absence of risk factors for atherosclerosis.

Raynaud's Syndrome

Raynaud's syndrome (RS) is characterized by episodic attacks of vasospasm resulting in the closure of small arteries and arterioles of the distal extremities in response to *cold* or *stress*. This exaggerated response causes a profound reduction in peripheral blood flow, which is abnormally slow to return. Mild pain, paresthesias, and numbness are frequent complaints, but severe pain is rare. Although the hands and fingers are most commonly affected, the toes, feet, and ears may be involved. The disease usually follows a benign course, but in long-standing cases, trophic changes may develop that lead to atrophy of the skin, subcutaneous tissue, and muscles.

PATHOPHYSIOLOGY. An episode of RS is classically described as occurring in three phases: pallor, cyanosis, and rubor. Pallor is caused by spasm of the palmar and digital vessels, with cessation of capillary perfusion. Cyanosis follows when the capillaries and venules dilate as a result of prolonged hypoxia, causing pooling of deoxygenated blood. The rubor is a consequence of the return of normal arterial blood flow into a dilated capillary bed. Most patients with RS do not experience this classic triphasic response but will report "cold hands" or episodes of pale or cyanotic fingertips.

Patients with RS may be divided into two distinct pathophysiologic groups—those with obstructive RS and those with spastic RS. Patients with *obstructive RS* typically have an underlying disorder with obstruction of the palmar and digital arteries, causing a significant reduction in digital arterial pressure. A normal vasoconstrictive response to cold is then sufficient to cause arterial closure. Patients with *spastic RS* have a normal digital arterial pressure at room temperature, but arterial closure occurs as a result of an *exaggerated,* cold-induced spasm.

Although the exact nature of this localized phenomenon remains unclear, abnormal platelet adhesiveness, increased blood viscosity, reduced red cell deformability and an imbalance in the production of prostacyclin and thromboxane have been implicated. Recent studies have suggested an altered adrenergic receptor function in patients with spastic RS. Patients with RS have an increased density and sensitivity of peripheral alpha-adrenoceptors in both the vessel wall and platelet membrane in addition to presynaptic beta-adrenoceptor hypersensitivity with a clinical response to beta-blockers.

CLINICAL PRESENTATION. Patients with RS can be categorized into two clinical entities: ***primary Raynaud's syndrome*** typically occurs in young, otherwise healthy women and accounts for 60% to 70% of all cases. It is thought to be caused by vasospasm and may become clinically evident at any time during the second or third decade of life. Episodes typically occur symmetrically, most often involve both hands and fingers (sparing the thumbs), and they usually last for 20 to 30 minutes. Most patients with primary RS have *mild* involvement of the feet and toes, but only 10% have primary lower extremity disease. Although one finger may be affected during an episode, it is more common for all the fingers to be involved, from the tips to the metacarpophalangeal joints. Tissue injury and necrosis are very uncommon with primary RS.

In ***secondary Raynaud's syndrome*** (Raynaud's phenomenon) an associated disorder is thought to be the cause of the patient's symptoms. All of these conditions produce spastic and/or obstructive arterial phenomena. Secondary RS should be considered in any patient with (1) early or late age of onset of Raynaud's attacks, (2) male sex, (3) asymmetric or painful attacks, (4) signs of tissue necrosis, or (5) presence of a coexisting disease. This secondary RS has been associated with scleroderma, systemic lupus erythematosus, dermatomyositis, and Sjögren's syndrome; often occlusive lesions occur in the small arteries within the hand.

DIAGNOSIS. A careful history and physical examination are necessary in the evaluation of patients with Raynaud's-type symptoms. Information should be sought from the patient about symptoms of large vessel occlusive disease, smoking and drug history, employment, exposure to trauma or frostbite, and history of malignancy. The skin of the hands and fingers should be carefully inspected for lesions or hyperkeratotic areas that would suggest healed ulcers. The results of a peripheral pulse examination should be carefully noted. The physical examination, however, is frequently unremarkable, and the diagnosis is usually made from the history alone.

A screening laboratory evaluation includes a complete blood count, platelet count, erythrocyte sedimentation rate, urinalysis, rheumatoid factor, and antinuclear antibody profile. Further tests may include antithrombin III, protein C, and protein S levels as well as anticardiolipin and lupus anticoagulant antibodies. In those patients in whom the diagnosis remains uncertain, the noninvasive vascular laboratory can be helpful in establishing a diagnosis of RS and distinguishing between a spastic or obstructive cause. A drop in baseline digital blood pressure in response to 5 minutes of hypothermia has an accuracy of 92% in the diagnosis of RS. Arteriography is usually reserved for patients with finger gangrene or ulceration or those with unilateral symptoms in which a proximal arterial lesion is suspected (Fig. 13-1).

TREATMENT. Most patients with RS have mild symptoms that respond to conservative treatment such as wearing gloves and avoiding cold temperatures and tobacco (see the box on p. 253). Cigarette smoking may produce a fall in temperature of 2° to 3° C in the fingertips of normal people. Patients who work in a cold environment may not improve until their occupational exposure is reduced. Patients with stress-related attacks may benefit from biofeedback or behavior modification therapy.

Patients with severe attacks that are not responsive to conservative therapy or those with tissue ischemia may require pharmacologic intervention, usually with calcium channel blockers. Nifedipine has been shown to improve digital blood flow in patients with RS, but the side effects of systemic vasodilation (headache, flushing, and dizziness) occur in about one third of patients. The incidence of side effects can be reduced by starting with small doses (5 mg twice a day) and increasing the dosage slowly until an effective response is achieved.

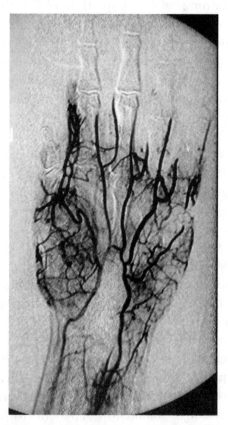

Fig. 13-1. Patient is a 32-year-old white female with severe isch-emia symptoms of the right hand. Angiogram following papav-erine injection shows occlusion of all digital vessels at the midfingers. (Courtesy Curtis W. Bakal, MD.)

Treatment Options for Raynaud's Syndrome

Cold Protection
Socks and gloves
Layered clothing

Behavior Modification
Avoidance of stress
Biofeedback (for stress-related disease)
Cessation of smoking
Avoidance of caffeine and other drugs

Vasodilation
Calcium channel blockers—nifedipine
Adrenergic blockers
    Alpha-blockers—thymoxamine
    Beta-blockers—propranolol
Serotonin antagonists—ketanserin
Prostaglandins and prostaglandin stimulators—iloprost
ACE inhibitors—captopril
Nitrates—transdermal glycerol trinitrate

Decreased Blood Viscosity
Platelet aggregation inhibitors
Plasmapheresis
Fibrinolysis
Increased red cell deformability
Volume expanders
Fish oils

Treatment of Underlying Condition
Surgical correction of anatomic abnormalities
Immunomodulating treatment for underlying connec-
    tive tissue disease

Thymoxamine, a competitive alpha$_1$-adrenoceptor blocker, causes vasodilation in some vascular beds while maintaining systemic vascular resistance. The explanation for this may be the 10:1 ratio of alpha$_1$:alpha$_2$ adrenoceptor activity in the skin. At doses of 40 to 80 mg four times a day there is symptomatic relief with minimal side effects. Other drugs currently being investigated include beta-blockers, transdermal PGE$_2$, and fish oils (see the box on p. 253).

Severe cases, particularly those with arterial occlusions or those in which there is ulceration or gangrene, are a challenge to clinicians and may require that the patient be hospitalized. Intra-arterial prostacyclin infusion frequently has immediate results, and the improvement may last for several months. In a small number of patients, a proximal cause of the arterial insufficiency will be discovered. Arteriosclerosis of the subclavian, axillary, or brachial arteries, the presence of emboli, or thoracic outlet syndrome are all indications for arterial reconstruction. Although cervicothoracic sympathectomy offers only temporary relief and is rarely used for Raynaud's syndrome, lumbar sympathectomy may be helpful in refractory lower extremity vasospasm.

In the treatment of finger gangrene resulting from secondary RS, conservative treatment should be the watchword. Careful hygiene, analgesic agents, and pharmacologic treatment will usually prevent the need for major digital amputations.

Buerger's Disease
(Thromboangiitis Obliterans)

In 1908 Leo Buerger published his observations and pathologic study of 11 amputated lower extremities, which both defined the disorder and served as a cornerstone for further study. Thromboangiitis obliterans (TAO) is a distinctive, segmental vasculitis of the small and medium-sized arteries of both the upper and lower extremities. It initially involves the distal vessels with proximal progression and typically occurs in men between the ages of 20 and 40 who have a history of heavy smoking. Although it was originally thought to occur only in men, several cases have been reported in women. While TAO affects all races, it is more common in Middle Eastern and Far Eastern people.

ETIOLOGIC FACTORS. While the cause of TAO remains unknown (some believe it is just an unusual form of early atherosclerosis), *all* patients with TAO are smokers, and the relationship of smoking to remissions and exacerbations of TAO has been demonstrated. It is likely, therefore, that TAO is an autoimmune reaction triggered by the use of tobacco. Evidence for this hypothesis includes an increased serum compliment factor (C4), antielastin and anticollagen antibodies, and cellular sensitivity to type I and III collagen. Tobacco glycoprotein antigen, which has been isolated from tobacco leaves, may be an important factor in the cell-mediated response to collagen.

CLINICAL PRESENTATION. The diagnosis of TAO should be considered in *any young smoker,* particularly if the upper extremities are involved, or if a history of migratory thrombophlebitis exists. The initial clinical manifestations are nonspecific: cold sensitivity, paresthesias, and skin color changes. Ulceration or gangrene occurs in 75% of patients and is associated with severe pain. The ischemic areas are usually well demarcated. Foot claudication, characteristic of TAO, is caused by infrapopliteal arterial occlusion. Recurrent superficial thrombophlebitis of the arm, lower leg, and foot develops in up to 50% of patients.

DIAGNOSIS. Atherosclerosis and autoimmune disease must be ruled out before a diagnosis of TAO is made. Although a diagnosis of TAO is usually made on the basis of histologic findings, the initial evaluation begins with a complete history and physical examination. Attention is paid to upper extremity symptoms, Raynaud's syndrome, superficial thrombophlebitis, and foot claudication. Accurate evaluation of peripheral pulses and evidence of ischemic changes at the tips of the fingers and toes must be documented. Serologic tests should be obtained to exclude autoimmune diseases. Noninvasive vascular laboratory evaluations are frequently helpful.

Arteriography in patients with TAO reveals segmental obstruction of medium-sized arteries of the calf and forearm. The characteristic "corkscrew" appearance of collateral vessels is seen in 25% of patients with this disease (Fig. 13-2).

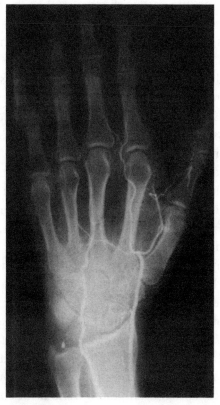

Fig. 13-2. Patient is a 41-year-old white male with a painful, nonhealing ulcer of the right hand. Angiogram of the upper extremity demonstrates occlusive disease of the digital vessels and reconstitution of the distal princeps pollicis artery.

TREATMENT. The clinical course of the patient with TAO is marked by exacerbations of rapidly worsening arterial insufficiency with severe ischemic pain. However, cessation of smoking will eliminate these exacerbations and will halt the progression of the disease process.

Medical treatment is aimed at increasing flow through the remaining patent vessels. Systemically administered vasodilators have little effect on collateral vessels; however, continuous intra-arterial administration of prostaglandin E_1 does produce maximal vasodilatation which is of benefit to patients with intractable ulceration. Thallium-201 has been of use in predicting the likelihood of healing an ischemic ulcer. Unlike patients with atherosclerotic disease, patients who undergo digital amputations heal *well*.

Sympathectomy and distal arterial reconstruction should be considered for patients with ulcers that do not heal. There is a higher incidence of graft failure in TAO compared with arteriosclerosis, but patency of the graft for several months is frequently sufficient to heal skin lesions. The use of free and pedicled omental grafts have also been successfully employed. When gangrene occurs, digital amputation should be considered.

Collagen Vascular Diseases

Vasculitis refers to an inflammatory process of the blood vessels with progressive intimal proliferation and thrombosis. Vasculitis may be idiopathic, primary, or may occur in association with other systemic diseases. Most current opinion relates the vasculitis to the deposition of immune complexes within the vessel wall.

POLYARTERITIS NODOSA. Polyarteritis nodosa (PAN) is a necrotizing vasculitis involving small and medium-sized muscular arteries. It is a rare disorder, with a mean age at onset of 45 years and a male to female ratio of 2.5:1. Involvement of the renal and visceral arteries with sparing of the pulmonary circulation is characteristic. The lesions are segmental and often involve branching points. Necrotizing vasculitis with fibrinoid necrosis of the vessel wall occurs in the acute phase of PAN, commonly resulting in microaneurysm formation.

Clinical presentation. Patients typically present with vague symptoms such as weakness, malaise, headache, abdominal pain, or myalgias. Renal involvement occurs in 85% of patients and most commonly manifests as ischemic changes in the glomeruli. The cutaneous manifestations of PAN, occurring in 40% of patients, include palpable purpura and ulceration. Cardiac involvement (congestive heart failure) is clinically apparent in one third of patients. Involvement of the gastrointestinal tract occurs in 45% of patients and presents as nausea, vomiting, and abdominal pain. Patients may also develop pancreatitis, intra-abdominal hemorrhage (6%), or bowel perforation (5%) as a result of their vasculitis.

Diagnosis. The diagnosis of PAN is made histologically. In the absence of tissue for biopsy, angiographic demonstration of involved vessels, particularly aneurysms of small and medium-sized arteries (renal, hepatic, and visceral) is usually sufficient to make the diagnosis. There are no diagnostic serologic tests for PAN. However, more than 75% of patients with PAN will have an elevated leukocyte count and erythrocyte sedimentation rate.

Treatment. The prognosis of untreated PAN is poor, with a 5-year survival rate of less than 15%. Favorable therapeutic results have been reported with the combination of prednisone and cyclophosphamide, which has resulted in up to a 90% remission rate.

TEMPORAL (GIANT CELL) ARTERITIS. Temporal or giant cell arteritis (GCA) is a vasculitis of medium- and large-sized arteries. It commonly affects the branches of the carotid artery, particularly the temporal arteries; however, systemic involvement may occur. Most cases of GCA occur after the age of 55. It is more common in women, and it is rare in black patients. The disease is characterized by fever, anemia, headaches, and a high erythrocyte sedimentation rate. The headaches do not follow a characteristic pattern and may be accompanied by scalp pain or jaw claudication. Ischemic optic neuritis, a complication of GCA, may lead to visual symptoms including sudden monocular or binocular blindness.

Polymyalgia rheumatica is present in over 50% of patients with GCA and is characterized by stiffness and myalgias of the neck, shoulder, lower back, or thigh. Clinical involvement of the large arteries of the extremities is rare in patients with GCA (<10%). Although stenosis or occlusion is frequently progressive and bilaterally symmetric, claudication with loss of distal pulses is the rule rather than limb-threatening ischemia. The upper extremity is more commonly involved.

The diagnosis of GCA is usually a clinical one when fever, anemia, a high erythrocyte sedimentation rate, and symptoms of polymyalgia rheumatica are present in an elderly patient. Biopsy of the temporal artery is performed to confirm the diagnosis. The most clinically abnormal site should be biopsied, and if there is no distinctly abnormal artery on examination, a longer (5 cm) segment of artery should be biopsied. GCA responds well to corticosteroid therapy. Treatment should begin with 40 to 60 mg of prednisone per day followed by a gradual tapering to 7.5 to 10 mg per day.

TAKAYASU'S ARTERITIS. Takayasu's arteritis (TA) was first described in 1908 by a Japanese ophthalmologist. It is an uncommon, chronic inflammatory arteriopathy of unknown causes. TA is characteristically a disease of young women between the ages of 10 and 40. TA typically involves the aorta and its major branches, with pulmonary artery involvement reported in approximately 50% of cases.

TA is divided into three groups: (1) disease limited to the aortic arch (30%), (2) disease limited to the descending aorta (10% to 15%), and (3) disease involving the entire aorta (60%). The clinical features of TA vary, making early diagnosis difficult. Initial symptoms may include fever, malaise, arthritis, anemia, weight loss, and arthralgias. Pericardial pain, tachycardia, and vomiting may occur. This initial phase may be followed by vessel inflammation, leading to stenosis or aneurysm formation. This may lead to vascular insufficiency of the upper extremities, presenting as arm claudication, paresthesias, or numbness. Patients will commonly have a pulse discrepancy of more than 30 mm Hg between the left and right arms. Less commonly, patients will have lower extremity claudication, which is distinguished from atherosclerotic disease by the absence of the usual risk factors in a young population. Physical findings usually include bruits or diminished pulses. Postural dizziness is common and reflects occlusive disease of the carotid or vertebrobasilar systems. Visual disturbances are present in 30% of these patients, while arthralgias are reported in 55%. Coronary artery disease, caused by ostial narrowing, may occur.

Rapid progression of the disease and death within 2 years of diagnosis occurs in approximately 10% of patients. Initial therapy mandates aggressive management of the acute inflammatory process with cortico-steroids and cyclophosphamide. Indications for operation depend on the site and severity of arterial involvement. Surgery for brachiocephalic trunk disease is rarely necessary and should be limited to patients with neurologic symptoms or severe upper extremity claudication. Operative indications for aneurysmal dilation of the aorta caused by TA are similar to that of atherosclerotic disease; however, surgery may be difficult during the active inflammatory stage. Aortic and renal artery procedures may be required for the management of hypertension. Splanchnic vessel involvement is common; however, it is rare for this to become clinically apparent as collateral flow to the viscera is usually extensive.

RHEUMATOID VASCULITIS. Rheumatoid vasculitis, a rare complication of rheumatoid arthritis (RA), occurs in two forms. Digital vasculitis, more commonly affecting men with a high rheumatoid factor titer, typically manifests with transient microinfarctions (<1 mm) and frequent recurrences. This entity is self-limiting and requires only conservative treatment. Less often, patients with RA develop a more active vasculitis of the small and medium-sized arteries that is indistinguishable from periarteritis nodosa. This occurs late in the course of RA in patients with advanced joint changes, cutaneous nodules, and a positive antinuclear antibody test. Cutaneous manifestations include ischemic ulcers, extensive digital gangrene, and palpable purpura. Most patients will have involvement of more than one extremity. Weight loss, pleuritis, pericarditis, mesenteric ischemia, and ocular inflammation have all been reported. Involvement of the gastrointestinal tract occurs in 10% of cases and may be an early manifestation of the disease.

Biopsy or angiography will frequently confirm the diagnosis. Treatment is directed towards the underlying disease process and includes the use of corticosteroids, D-penicillamine, or cyclophosphamide.

SYSTEMIC LUPUS ERYTHEMATOSUS. Systemic lupus erythematosus (SLE) occurs primarily in young women. Arthritis, nephritis, pericarditis, cerebritis, and lymphadenopathy occur in varying combinations. Raynaud's syndrome is seen in approximately 20% of patients with SLE and may precede other manifestations of the disease. More than 20% of patients with SLE will develop dermal vasculitis with skin nodules or ulceration. Although abdominal pain is a frequent complaint of patients with SLE, clinically significant mesenteric vasculitis remains uncommon. Mesenteric ischemia, although infrequent, is a devastating complication of SLE with a mortality of over 50%.

The lupus anticoagulant antibody found in 5% to 10% of cases is associated with thrombosis of arteries and veins. Arterial involvement most commonly occurs in, but is not limited to, the digital arteries. If revascularization is performed, appropriate postoperative anticoagulation with heparin and coumadin must be maintained.

Fibromuscular Dysplasia

Fibromuscular dysplasia (FMD) represents a heterogeneous group of nonatherosclerotic, noninflammatory diseases of small and medium-sized arteries. The principal forms include intimal fibroplasia, medial hyperplasia, and medial fibroplasia. The most common form, medial fibrodysplasia, accounts for 70% to 95% of all fibromuscular lesions and most commonly involves the renal (60% to 75%) and carotid (25% to 30%) arteries. Venous involvement is rare.

Although the pathogenesis of FMD is incompletely understood, humoral, mechanical, and genetic factors as well as mural ischemia may play a role in its development. Young white women are most commonly affected. Patients may be asymptomatic or present with renovascular hypertension, stroke, abdominal angina, or claudication. The natural history of FMD is usually benign, with progression of the disease occurring in only a minority of patients.

FMD is the underlying cause in 20% to 50% of patients with renovascular hypertension. In children and young women with renovascular hypertension, FMD is responsible for the majority of cases. It has been postulated that FMD may be secondary to trauma or stretching of the renal artery. The right kidney, which is the more mobile and whose artery is more frequently stretched during pregnancy, is affected 85% of the time. Renal artery aneurysms are frequently present and may lead to thrombosis or embolization.

FMD should be suspected in any patient with the sudden onset of hypertension, particularly in women of childbearing age. Patients typically have a sustained elevation of the diastolic blood pressure which is resistant to medical therapy. The diagnosis of FMD can be made with a high degree of accuracy on the basis of its angiographic appearance. It usually involves the *middle* or *distal* segments of the renal arteries with smooth, concentric lesions and the "string-of-beads" appearance is characteristic. In contrast, atherosclerotic lesions are usually eccentric and located within 1 cm of the orifice of the main renal artery with atherosclerotic changes in the aorta.

There are currently three therapeutic approaches to FMD of the renal arteries: vascular reconstruction, percutaneous transluminal angioplasty (PTA), and nephrectomy. Vascular reconstruction techniques include revascularization, operative arterial dilation, or autotransplantation. PTA has been more successful with "string-of-beads" stenoses than with focal lesions. The results of both surgical treatment and PTA are best with unilateral FMD with "cure rates" ranging from 38% to 85%. Nephrectomy is indicated when revascularization has failed or is technically impossible or the kidney is nonfunctional. In patients with cerebrovascular FMD, surgical intervention should be reserved for patients with progressive cerebral ischemia. Graduated intraluminal dilation is the method of choice for FMD of the extracranial arteries with a low morbidity, mortality, and recurrence rate.

BIBLIOGRAPHY

Brotzu G, Falchi S, Mannu B, Montisci R, Petruzzo P, Staico R. The importance of presynaptic beta receptors in Raynaud's disease. J Vasc Surg 9:767, 1989.

Conn DL. Rheumatic Disease Clinics of North America: Vasculitic Syndromes. Philadelphia: WB Saunders, 1990.

Cooke ED, Nicolaides AN. Raynaud's syndrome: Thymoxamine, iloprost, and ACE inhibitors are among the effective treatments now available. Br Med J 300:553-555, 1990.

Edwards JM, Porter JM. Associated diseases with Raynaud's syndrome. Vasc Med Rev 1:51-58, 1990.

Fauci AS, Haynes BF, Katz P. The spectrum of vasculitis: Clinical, pathologic, immunologic, and therapeutic considerations. Ann Intern Med 89:660-676, 1978.

Lagneau P, Michel JB, Vuong PN. Surgical treatment of Takayasu's disease. Ann Surg 205:157-166, 1987.

Luscher TF, Lie JT, Stanson AW, Houser AW, Hollier LH, Sheps SG. Arterial fibromuscular dysplasia. Mayo Clin Proc 62:931-952, 1987.

Ohta T, Shinonoya S. Fate of the ischaemic limb in Buerger's disease. Br J Surg 75:259-262, 1988.

Papa M, Bass A, Adar R, Halperin Z, Schneiderman J, Becker CG, Brautbar H, Mozes E. Autoimmune mechanisms in thromboangiitis obliterans (Buerger's disease): The role of tobacco antigen and the major histocompatibility complex. Surgery 111:527-531, 1992.

14

Diseases of the Venous and Lymphatic Systems

Amit V. Patel

Venous thrombosis, valvular incompetence, and pulmonary embolism are the three most common manifestations of venous disease in the lower extremities. Knowledge of the anatomy allows for a greater understanding of the disease entities discussed in this chapter.

Lower Extremity Venous Anatomy

The superficial venous system consists of the greater and lesser saphenous veins, which are located on the anteromedial and posterior aspects of the lower extremity, respectively. These veins are superficial to the fascia and have multiple valves. They communicate, via perforators, with the deep venous system and account for approximately 10% of the venous flow in normal individuals.

The named veins of the deep venous system include the superficial and deep femoral, popliteal, anterior and posterior tibial, and peroneal veins—all of which accompany their respective arteries. The veins below the knee are often paired and account for 90% of the venous return of the lower extremity.

The superficial and deep systems are connected by the perforating veins, which traverse the fascia. Perhaps the most important anatomic feature of normal veins is the presence of valves; they direct flow in a cephalad direction as well as from the superficial to the deep systems with the assistance of muscular movement.

Venous Thrombosis

Venous thrombosis is a common problem that is potentially life threatening. It is best treated prophylactically, but when it is diagnosed it must be treated aggressively. The pathogenesis of venous thrombosis has changed very little since Virchow first described the triad of venous stasis, epithelial injury, and hypercoagulability in 1856.

> **Virchow's Triad: Fundamental Causes of Venous Thrombosis**
>
> Venous stasis
> Epithelial injury
> Hypercoagulability

Venous stasis is clearly a problem in an immobile post-operative patient. Any other risk factor that reduces flow, such as extrinsic compression from masses or valvular incompetence, can result in venous thrombosis. Epithelial injury may occur after trauma or surgery. A hypercoagulable state exists in the postoperative period as well as in patients with a malignancy, smoking history, congenital anticoagulant deficiency, or who are pregnant or use exogenous estrogen.

DIAGNOSIS. Venous thrombosis is classified and treated according to the system that is involved. ***Deep venous thrombosis*** (DVT) is a common problem that requires aggressive treatment to prevent serious complications. Superficial venous thrombosis, more commonly seen in outpatients, usually responds well to conservative therapy unless it involves the greater saphenous vein in the thigh.

The diagnosis of DVT on the basis of history and physical examination is correct in only 50% of cases. The diagnosis must be considered in any patient who has unilateral swelling, calf pain or tenderness, calf pain on dorsiflexion (Homan's sign), or a tender, palpable cord in the popliteal or femoral region. Fifty percent of DVTs are "silent" and the patient is asymptomatic. Superficial thrombophlebitis usually presents with a tender, palpable cord in the course of the greater or lesser saphenous veins.

The standard diagnostic method has been venography; however, improvements in duplex ultrasonography have changed this. Venography involves injection of a contrast medium into a vein in the foot, with subsequent radiographic visualization of the venous system. It is invasive and the potential complications include contrast-induced allergic reaction and thrombophlebitis at the site of injection.

Doppler ultrasound can be used to detect flow in all of the veins of the lower extremity (see Chapter 3). The venous flow is identified by listening for the arterial signal and identifying the venous signal adjacent to it. Augmentation of flow with expiration and a slowing of flow with inspiration should be present. Diagnostically, the flow should be augmented by compressing the lower extremity at various points distal to the probe. A patent venous system will produce an increase in the flow, whereas a venous obstruction will inhibit augmentation of flow. This is a simple and rapid method for diagnosing complete occlusions and is accurate in 85% of cases. However, it is operator dependent and requires experience with the technique. Partial occlusions are often missed using this Doppler technique, so that other modalities may be required for identification.

Duplex ultrasonography has replaced venography in many centers as the standard method for detecting venous thrombosis. It combines Doppler flow detection with ultrasound imaging of the clot and vessel. The duplex examination can be used to assess the iliac veins and inferior vena cava as well as the veins of the lower extremity. However, the accuracy of duplex ultrasound is significantly reduced in the below-knee venous system.

A less frequently used noninvasive examination is the radioactively labeled fibrinogen uptake test. This study documents the uptake of circulating radioactive fibrinogen into newly forming thrombi. The major drawback to this test is its high sensitivity, thereby identifying a large number of subclinical thrombi that do not require treatment. It will *not* detect an old thrombosis, and therefore, with its high sensitivity and a 12- to 24-hour period required to perform the test, it is no longer commonly used for screening patients suspected of having DVT.

TREATMENT

Thrombophlebitis. Superficial thrombophlebitis is diagnosed primarily on the basis of the physical examination. A palpable tender cord along the course of the greater or lesser saphenous vein is present in addition to mild erythema of the skin. It is usually a benign and self-limited condition. However, suppurative thrombophlebitis or thrombosis extending *to* the saphenofemoral junction requires early, aggressive therapy. Excision of a suppurative thrombophlebitic vein is mandatory and must be accompanied by a course of intravenous antibiotic therapy. When thrombus in the greater saphenous vein extends above the knee, high ligation of the saphenous vein is indicated. Anticoagulation therapy is instituted until the patient can be brought to the operating room to prevent the extension of thrombus into the deep system, with subsequent pulmonary emboli.

In the absence of these complications, superficial thrombophlebitis can be treated with anti-inflammatory medications, heat, and other symptomatic treatments. Exercise and activity should be encouraged, with follow-up clinical and duplex examination within 72 hours to ensure that the thrombosis has not progressed. Proximal progression to the saphenofemoral junction may occur, but propagation through perforators into the deep system is extremely unusual. In addition, conversion from aseptic to suppurative thrombophlebitis is unlikely unless the initial thrombosis resulted from injection or invasive trauma.

When fever, chills, and leukocytosis are present, suppurative thrombophlebitis should be suspected. This septic thrombophlebitis is most commonly caused by *Staphylococcus aureus* and requires prompt treatment to prevent systemic complications. Intravenous antibiotics and excision of the affected vein are mandatory.

Deep-vein thrombosis. The objectives of treatment for DVT are to prevent formation of additional thrombi, inhibit propagation of existing thrombi, and minimize damage to the venous valves. Most important, however, is the prevention of pulmonary emboli. Five percent of patients with DVT will have pulmonary emboli despite adequate treatment. In 25% of patients with untreated DVT, pulmonary emboli will occur, and a substantial number of these will have fatal outcomes.

When DVT is *suspected*, immediate anticoagulation therapy should be instituted. Confirmatory tests are obtained when available; however, full anticoagulation should not await the results of these studies. If a contraindication to anticoagulation therapy exists (for example, a recent surgical procedure, malignancy, or active hemorrhage), therapy should be *delayed* until a definitive diagnosis is established. Immediate anticoagulation is achieved by bolus intravenous administration of heparin (5000 to 10,000 U) followed by a continuous infusion of heparin solution to maintain the partial thromboplastin time at 1.5 to 2 times the control value. The platelet count must be monitored daily to allow early identification of heparin-induced thrombocytopenia.

Subsequent conversion to a course of oral anticoagulation therapy (with warfarin) is begun 3 to 7 days after full heparinization is achieved. The dose of warfarin is regulated with an objective of maintaining the prothrombin time at 1.5 to 2 times the control value. The duration of therapy should be at least 3 to 6 months to allow for recanalization and collateral formation. Serial duplex ultrasonography examinations should be performed to evaluate progression or resolution of the thrombosis.

The use of thrombolytic agents such as urokinase and streptokinase has been advocated for the treatment of significant DVT. Although the long-term efficacy of such treatment is unclear, there may be a role for this treatment modality. The thrombolytic agent is administered through a peripheral vein, and the levels of fibrinogen and products of fibrinolysis are carefully monitored. Although the incidence of bleeding complications is increased, it appears that long-term post-thrombotic sequelae can be reduced.

Alternative therapy methods must be sought when anticoagulation therapy is contraindicated or in patients who develop pulmonary emboli while receiving adequate anticoagulation treatment. Placement of an inferior vena cava (IVC) filter will prevent the embolization of clot originating from the lower extremities. The majority of fatal pulmonary emboli originate in the pelvic vessels and IVC; therefore the presence of thrombus loosely adherent to the vessel wall ("free-floating") is another indication for placement of an IVC filter. The most commonly used device is the Greenfield filter—an intraluminal, cone-shaped filter—placed percutaneously via the femoral or jugular veins. Its placement in the infrarenal IVC is confirmed fluoroscopically. Alternatives to the Greenfield filter include other intraluminal devices and the use of caval clips and IVC ligation. These latter two procedures require operations and carry a greater risk of subsequent venous insufficiency; therefore they are seldom used today.

Thrombi involving the iliofemoral venous system often produce the most dramatic manifestations. There can be massive swelling, pain, and tenderness of the lower extremity. *Phlegmasia cerulea dolens* is a severe form of iliofemoral thrombosis that causes an obstruction to venous outflow. This is characterized by cyanosis, which can rarely progress to gangrene. *Phlegmasia alba dolens* is another variant of iliofemoral thrombosis characterized by arterial spasm and a pale, cool leg with diminished pulses. Venous thrombectomy of the common femoral vein with postoperative anticoagulation should be considered in these circumstances. In approximately two thirds of these patients venous occlusion recurs postoperatively, so the value of thrombectomy alone is unproven. However, the addition of an arteriovenous fistula improves patency and has been recommended by some investigators.

PROPHYLAXIS. Prophylactic treatment is recommended in patients who are at high risk for DVT.

Risk Factors for Venous Thrombosis

Immobility	Polycythemia
Obesity	Anticoagulant deficiency
Smoking	Pregnancy
Trauma	Estrogen use
Malignancy	

Mechanical methods currently used are pneumatic compression devices and antiembolism stockings. Drugs for prophylaxis include warfarin, heparin, and dextran. It is generally agreed that low-dose heparin, warfarin, and pneumatic compression devices are equivalent in efficacy and all reduce the incidence of venous thrombosis in high risk-patients.

Varicose Veins

Varicose veins are elongated, tortuous, dilated vessels. They most commonly occur in the lower extremity but can be found in other parts of the body, such as the scrotum (varicocele), esophagus (esophageal varices), and anal canal (hemorrhoids). Varicose veins are classified as primary or secondary. Primary varicose veins are not associated with deep venous pathologic conditions, whereas secondary varicose veins are caused by deep venous insufficiency or obstruction. The distinction between primary and secondary varicose veins is not always obvious.

The cause of primary varicose veins may be obscure. The fundamental abnormality is sequential incompetence of the valves of the saphenous or perforator veins. Secondary varicosities occur as a result of previous trauma or DVT with subsequent valvular incompetency. Regardless of the cause, reversal of flow occurs with subsequent development of varicosities.

Patients with symptomatic varicose veins usually complain of painful, swollen, or "heavy-feeling" legs or bleeding from varicosities. Others may simply dislike the appearance for cosmetic reasons. The initial evaluation for valvular competency involves the Trendelenburg test. The patient is placed supine with elevation of the affected leg. A tourniquet is placed on the upper thigh to compress the greater saphenous vein, thereby simulating a competent saphenofemoral junction. The patient stands with the tourniquet in place, and the varices (which had emptied) are observed for 30 seconds. Normally the superficial veins will fill slowly, but with incompetence of the perforators, the varicosities will fill rapidly while the tourniquet is on. Rapid filling of the varicose veins that occurs following removal of the tourniquet suggests incompetence of the saphenofemoral junction. Duplex ultrasonography is useful in documenting the incompetence of the saphenofemoral valves as well as those of the perforating veins.

Treatment of varicosities depends on the severity and cause as well as the patient's lifestyle, medical status, and wishes. Current management employs compression stockings, sclerotherapy, high ligation of the saphenous vein, vein stripping, and stab avulsion of varicosities. The type of treatment depends on the extent of disease as well as the anatomic location.

Elastic support, along with periodic exercise and elevation, is the treatment of choice for most patients. Excellent relief of symptoms is achieved in most instances. Sclerotherapy injections induce a dense fibrotic reaction and result in obliteration of the vein. This is best reserved for "spider" intracutaneous veins and small varicosities and produces good cosmetic results. The slight chance of extravasation of the sclerosing agent, with unsightly skin staining and ulceration, must be recognized before recommending this technique. Surgical therapy involves removal of the varices and ligation of incompetent veins. Vein stripping, a procedure that is currently done less frequently to preserve the greater saphenous vein for bypass surgery, is performed by entering the saphenous vein at the ankle and passing an intraluminal vein stripper proximally to the divided saphenous vein in the groin. The vein is then removed and compressive dressings applied. When a diagnosis of an incompetent saphenofemoral valve is made, high ligation of the saphenous vein is recommended. This is performed through a groin incision and the saphenous vein is divided at its origin at the common femoral vein. This can be accompanied by stab avulsions of the varicosities in the lower leg performed through separate small incisions. Stab avulsion is performed when there are numerous tributaries and perforators. Varicosities recur after surgical therapy in approximately 10% of patients.

Chronic Venous Insufficiency and Venous Stasis Disease

Chronic venous insufficiency is a result of persistent venous obstruction. This can be caused by the incomplete recanalization of previously thrombosed veins or, more commonly, valvular destruction.

The sustained high pressure, along with a disordered interstitial fluid clearance, results in the ***postphlebitic syndrome***. This syndrome consists of edema, stasis dermatitis, and ulceration. The edema involves the distal extremity and is usually the first manifestation of chronic venous insufficiency. Dermatitis and hyperpigmentation are caused by hemosiderin deposition in macrophages from extravasated red blood cells. Ulceration is the most common reason for which patients seek medical attention. Approximately half of all venous ulcers are associated with incompetent perforating veins in the region of the ankle. Stasis ulcers are most commonly located near the medial malleolus and often develop after minor trauma or infection.

When the history and physical examination suggest venous disease and further workup is necessary, noninvasive venous studies are obtained. The examiner must be assured by pulse examination or noninvasive testing that there is no arterial component to the ulceration. Venous duplex scanning documents venous patency and can quantitate valvular reflux in the deep and superficial systems. Impedance plethysmography is another noninvasive method to quantitate the degree of venous obstruction. Venographic evaluation may also be used to determine the degree of patency of the venous system, the presence of perforator incompetence, and the extent of collateral venous return.

The goal of therapy for venous insufficiency is the control of high venous pressures and the prevention of edema. This is accomplished in most patients with elastic compression stockings or may involve daily use of sequential compression devices.

A variety of dressings exist for the treatment of venous stasis ulcers. The most common of these is the medicated gelocast dressing (Unna's boot). The dressing is reapplied every 1 to 2 weeks until the ulcer has healed. Following satisfactory healing of the ulcer, the use of the elastic compression stockings is begun. Larger ulcers may require hospitalization for bed rest, leg elevation, and aggressive wound care.

If ulcers are large or are not responsive to conservative treatment, surgical therapy is indicated. Skin grafts may be applied to granulating ulcers or directly after excision of the ulcer. Recurrences are common if the underlying cause of the venous hypertension is not addressed. Surgical therapy includes greater saphenous vein stripping and ligation of the perforators in the region of the ulcer.

Other surgical alternatives include ligation of the perforators without stripping. The *Cockett procedure* involves ligation of the perforators behind the medial malleolus as they enter the deep fascia of the leg. The *Linton procedure* is similar except that it requires more extensive dissection and ligation of the perforators in a subfascial plane.

Venous reconstruction with bypass of an occluded iliac or femoral vein, valve repair, or transplantation has been reported. However, these procedures are not widely used. Their proponents claim that they return the venous system to a better level of function and that they allow healing of stasis ulceration in selected patients.

Lymphedema

Lymphedema is the collection of interstitial fluid. This is caused by obstruction of the lymphatics due to congenital or acquired causes. *Primary lymphedema* is an abnormality of the lymphatics *superficial* to the deep muscle fascia. Approximately 50% of patients with primary lymphedema develop bilateral involvement. Congenital lymphedema is usually present at birth but can occur later in life and is called *lymphedema praecox*. Lymphedema praecox is predominantly a disease of females and begins during puberty and adolescence. The initial symptoms are usually swelling of the ankle or foot, which worsens with activity. It is progressive and will eventually involve the entire leg. *Milroy's disease* is a hereditary form of lymphedema that usually presents at birth, but in a small percentage may present after the age of 35 (*lymphedema tarda*). Primary lymphedema is caused by hypoplasia, dilatation, or aplasia of the superficial lymphatics. This results in a functional obstruction with increased lymphatic pressures. As the lymphatic vessels enlarge, their valves become incompetent and stasis occurs. Stasis causes interstitial fluid to increase, resulting in fibrosis with worsening edema.

Secondary lymphedema results from an identifiable cause. Malignant obstruction of lymphatics is seen in prostatic cancer and lymphoma. Surgical procedures such as radical mastectomies or pelvic dissections cause lymphedema when lymphatics are divided. Filarial infections of the lymphatics cause obstruction and valvular disruption, with subsequent lymphedema in areas of the world with this parasite.

Complications of lymphedema include thickened skin, edema, cellulitis, and recurrent lymphangitis. Patients with lymphangitis present with tender, swollen, erythematous extremities. The infection spreads via the lymphatic vessels and produces characteristic red streaking from the site of infection proximally. Streptococcus is the most commonly isolated organism.

Lymphangiosarcomas are rare complications of lymphedema. They arise from the lymphatic endothelial cells and are almost always associated with a prior history of lymphedema. The tumor appears as multiple red, blue, or purple macular or papular lesions in the skin or subcutaneous tissue. They may form a larger mass that can ulcerate. Lymphangiosarcoma spreads very rapidly and has a poor prognosis.

TREATMENT. The goal of treatment is to control the edema and prevent recurrent infections. The majority of patients can be managed nonoperatively with custom compression stockings and weight loss if they are obese. Other measures to reduce the edema, such as dietary sodium restriction and extremity elevation, are also necessary. Intermittent compression devices are helpful in patients with mild to moderate disease. Patients are instructed to avoid minor trauma, since they are at an increased risk of developing cellulitis and lymphangitis. If infections recur, prophylactic antibiotics are recommended. This is a chronic condition, and patient education is essential for long-term compliance.

A small number of patients require surgical correction. This is usually indicated in patients who are physically impaired, have recurrent infections or lymphangiosarcoma, or those who wish cosmetic correction. Extensive staged removal of subcutaneous tissue and skin can be effective, although it requires two or more major procedures.

Procedures to increase the lymphatic drainage have been advocated. The ***Thompson procedure*** involves implanting flaps of beveled skin below the muscles and along the medial and lateral aspects of the leg to allow the superficial lymphatics to drain into the deep system. Results are equivocal (at best), and such operations as well as microsurgical procedures on the lymphatic vessels are not widely used and are yet to be proven effective.

BIBLIOGRAPHY

Bernstein EF, ed. Noninvasive Diagnostic Techniques in Vascular Disease, 5th ed. St. Louis: CV Mosby, 1993.

Browse NL, Burnand, KG, Thomas ML, eds. Diseases of the Veins: Pathology, Diagnosis and Treatment. New York: Arnold Publishing, 1988.

Hirsch J, Genton E, Hull R. Venous Thromboembolism. New York: Grune & Stratton, 1981.

Strandness DE Jr, Thiele BL. Selected Topics in Venous Disorders: Pathophysiology, Diagnosis and Treatment. New York: Futura Publishing, 1981.

15

Lower Extremity Amputation

Alan M. Dietzek • Larry A. Scher

Amputation is one of the oldest known surgical procedures. However, it was not until the mid-1500s that Ambroise Paré described the surgical techniques that are still in use today. Although often considered a destructive procedure, amputation, when appropriately performed, offers enormous potential for rehabilitation in most patients.

Indications for Amputation

The timing of amputation depends on the patient's clinical presentation. Emergent amputation is indicated for traumatic injuries, overwhelming infections, and, in rare instances, acute ischemia. An elective amputation may be performed in patients presenting with tissue necrosis who are not candidates for revascularization or in patients with malignancies.

Emergent Amputation

TRAUMA. Amputation is performed less frequently following injury of an extremity because of improvements in replantation surgery. However, severe crush injury remains a common indication for amputation. The level of amputation is dictated by the location of the injury. If the viability of the tissue surrounding the injury is questionable, an open amputation should be performed. This allows continuous assessment of the wound and subsequent revision to a closed stump. The goal of amputation is the preservation of length to facilitate rehabilitation. Preservation of the knee joint facilitates ambulation.

INFECTION. Tissue necrosis with superimposed infection (purulence, malodor, cellulitis) is often called *wet gangrene* and is a true surgical emergency. Operative debridement and amputation are the mainstays of therapy. Following amputation, the skin is left open ("guillotine" amputation) to allow drainage of residual infection. A definitive or closed amputation in this setting is associated with a higher rate of stump infection.

ACUTE ISCHEMIA. Acute lower extremity ischemia may result in irreversible soft tissue injury and necrosis. Urgent amputation is necessary when the acutely ischemic limb produces extensive muscle necrosis and systemic toxicity. Calf swelling, tenderness, muscle rigidity, and myoglobinuria are all signs of myonecrosis.

Elective Amputation

CHRONIC ISCHEMIA. Most patients with chronic limb-threatening ischemia are candidates for revascularization. Patients with severe organic mental syndrome or extensive necrosis or infection extending proximal to the tarsal bones should be considered for primary amputation. Additionally, patients with threatened limbs who have had multiple, previous failed attempts at limb salvage may be candidates for elective amputation.

Determination of Amputation Level

A variety of objective methods are presently used for determining the most distal level at which an amputation will heal. Clinical judgment alone can be used to successfully predict healing in approximately 80% of below-knee amputations and 90% of above-knee amputations. The presence of a palpable pulse proximal to the amputation level is an excellent predictor of successful amputation. The ability to heal an inframalleolar amputation is difficult to predict. Pulse examination accompanied by noninvasive testing may be beneficial.

SEGMENTAL BLOOD PRESSURE AND PULSE VOLUME RECORDINGS. *Segmental blood pressure* measured by a Doppler device and *pulse volume recordings* (PVRs) are the most commonly performed noninvasive vascular tests. Although their predictive value regarding healing of an amputation has been questioned, the absence of pulsatile blood flow, as determined by PVR tracings, is associated with a high rate of failure of forefoot amputations.

SKIN BLOOD FLOW TESTING. *Laser Doppler velocimetry, local skin fluorescence,* and *isotope measurements* are all used to quantitate cutaneous blood flow. These methods have all been reported to be of value in determining the level of amputation.

Magnetic resonance (MR) limb blood flow scanning allows assessment of whole-limb perfusion and measures blood flow through individual vessels. Further data must be obtained before the role of the MR scanner in determination of amputation level can be assessed.

SKIN TEMPERATURE MEASUREMENT. Clinical assessment of skin temperature is a subjective and unreliable means to determine extremity amputation level. Thermographic mapping is an objective means of ascertaining skin temperature which has correlated well with skin blood flow.

Surgical Techniques of Amputation

TOE AMPUTATION. A circular skin incision is made near the base of the toe (Fig. 15-1, *A*). Care should be taken to bevel the scalpel blade inward at the interdigital areas so there is no injury to the surrounding digits. The incision is brought through all tissue planes until the bone surface is scored circumferentially. A periosteal elevator is used to strip the periosteum for a short distance cephalad. The phalanx is then divided distal to the metatarsophalangeal joint using a bone cutter. Additional bone is removed using a rongeur, and a file or rasp is used to smooth the cut edge. One must prevent the metatarsal bone capsule from being exposed, because healing will not occur over this avascular surface. It is important that the cut edge of skin close over the phalanx without tension. The decision to close the skin (using interrupted monofilament sutures in a vertical mattress technique [Fig. 15-1, *B*]) is made with regard to the presence or absence of infection.

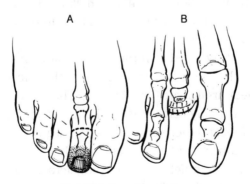

Fig. 15-1. Toe amputation.

RAY AMPUTATION. Tissue necrosis or infection that extends to the metatarsophalangeal crease is an indication for a ray amputation. A circular skin incision is made at the metatarsophalangeal crease (Fig. 15-2, *A*). The toe is amputated as described earlier, and a bone rongeur is used to remove any remaining phalangeal bone. A small periosteal elevator is used to free the metatarsal head from the attached tendons. The metatarsal head is carefully excised using a rongeur, and exposed tendons are pulled taut and divided as proximally as possible. After irrigation, the wound may be closed using interrupted monofilament sutures in a vertical mattress technique (Fig. 15-2, *B*). Ray amputation of the great toe requires a modified skin incision (Fig. 15-3, *A*) with a similar skin closure (Fig. 15-3, *B*).

TRANSMETATARSAL AMPUTATION. A transmetatarsal amputation is performed when gangrene extends slightly beyond the metatarsophalangeal crease. The plantar skin must be viable to be used in the creation of a posterior flap.

A slightly arced skin incision is made on the dorsum of the foot 5 to 10 mm distal to the midpoint of the metatarsal shafts (Fig. 15-4, *A*). The incision is extended halfway across the medial and lateral aspects of the foot and then gently curved 90 degrees. The incision is continued to the metatarsophalangeal crease, where it is completed by extension across the plantar surface of the foot. The incision is carried down to the

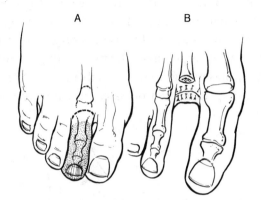

Fig. 15-2. Ray amputation.

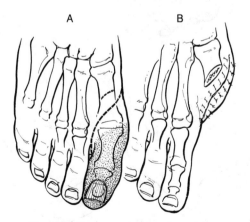

Fig. 15-3. Ray amputation of great toe.

level of the bones, and the metatarsals are divided proximal to the skin incision using either a bone cutter or oscillating saw (Fig. 15-4, *B*). The bone edges are flattened and smoothed and the tendons are divided as proximally as possible. The plantar flap is trimmed sharply, preserving a layer of subcutaneous fat. The plantar flap is rotated dorsally, and interrupted ab-

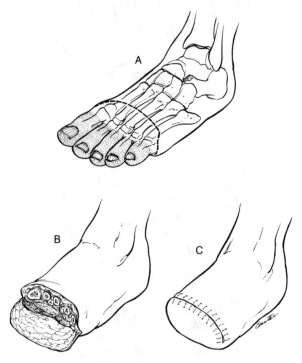

Fig. 15-4. Transmetatarsal amputation.

sorbable sutures are used to close the subcutaneous tissues. The skin is closed with interrupted monofilament sutures using the vertical mattress technique (Fig. 15-4, *C*).

SYME'S AMPUTATION. Syme's amputation (ankle disarticulation) has been advocated because it enhances rehabilitation potential. The dorsal incision is made anterior to the ankle crease starting at a point distal to the medial malleolus and extending to the lateral malleolus (Fig. 15-5, *A*). The incision is then carried posteriorly in a straight line on both sides and continued straight across the plantar surface of the foot anterior to the heel pad. This incision is carried down through the sole as well as on both sides to the calcaneus bone. The posterior tibial artery provides

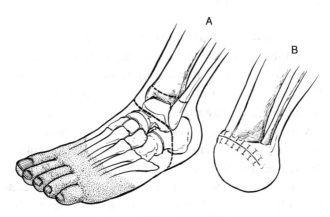

Fig. 15-5. Syme's amputation.

the blood supply to the heel and is therefore ligated distal to its bifurcation into the medial and lateral tarsal branches. The dorsal incision is brought down to the talus bone anterior to the ankle joint; the anterior tibial artery is ligated as necessary. The tendons are divided, allowing greater exposure of the talotibial joint by permitting plantar flexion of the foot. The joint capsule is then entered and the medial and lateral collateral ligaments are divided so that the talus may be disarticulated. The calcaneus is dissected from its soft tissue attachments without injuring the heel pad. The distal ends of both the tibia and fibula are cut with a saw and smoothed with a bone file. The heel flap is rotated anteriorly and the fascia is sutured to the deep fascia over the tibia. The skin is then closed using interrupted vertical mattress monofilament sutures (Fig. 15-5, *B*).

BELOW-KNEE AMPUTATION. Preservation of the knee joint, as in a below-knee amputation, is vital to facilitate transfer, even in bedridden patients. Although below-knee amputation may be performed by several methods, we advocate creation of a long posterior myocutaneous flap. The ideal level of tibial bone transection is approximately 12 cm below the tibial tuberosity. The anterior skin incision is made 1 cm distal to this point (Fig. 15-6, *A*) and continued medially and laterally to a point 1 cm posterior to the edge of the tibia and fibula, respectively. The incisions are angled as shown in Fig. 15-6, *A,* and extended distally for a distance between one third and one half the circumference of the leg as measured at the level of the proximal incision. A gently arced skin incision connects the medial and lateral incisions posteriorly. The greater and lesser saphenous veins are divided between silk ties, and the sural nerve is transected as high as possible to avoid painful neuromas in the stump. Division of the muscles of the anterior compartment will identify the anterior tibial neurovascular bundle, which is suture ligated. The remaining musculature is carefully dissected from the bony attachments, and the tibia is scored circumferentially with electrocautery. A laparotomy pad, moistened and passed behind the tibia, is used to strip the periosteum cephalad on all sides. The tibia is divided 2 cm proximal to the skin with the use of a pneumatic or hand saw. The tibia is then beveled at a 45-degree angle by cutting its anterior surface and carefully filing its edges smooth. The fibula is dissected in a similar manner; however, it is cut approximately 2 cm proximal to the level of the tibia transection. The posterior musculature is now exposed and the posterior tibial and peroneal neurovascular bundles are divided (Fig. 15-6, *B*). The remaining muscles are then divided using a large amputation (Lipson) knife (Fig. 15-6, *C* and *D*). Soleal veins may require suture ligature to ensure hemostasis. Often it is necessary to thin the posterior flap by either beveling the musculature or removing the soleus muscle. The

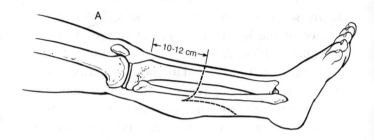

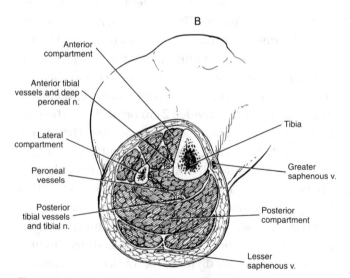

Fig. 15-6. A, Skin incision for below-knee amputation. **B,** Cross-sectional view of leg at level of skin incision. **C** and **D,** Creating posterior flap using a Lipson knife. **E,** Completed amputation with skin approximated musing vertical mattress sutures.

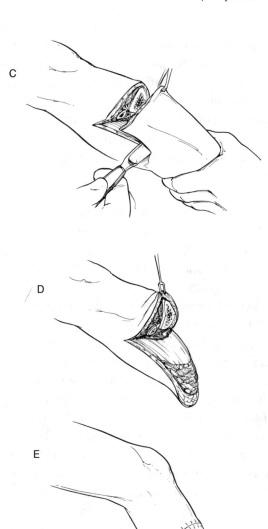

wound is irrigated with an antibiotic solution to remove all debris. The fascia of the anterior and posterior flaps are approximated with multiple interrupted absorbable sutures. Occasionally, placement of a closed-suction drain may be desirable. The skin is closed with either skin staples or monofilament sutures (Fig. 15-6, *E*), which are removed approximately 3 weeks after surgery.

ABOVE-KNEE AMPUTATION. Patients who are not candidates for a below-knee amputation because of infection, ischemia, or whose general condition precludes rehabilitation should be considered for an above-knee amputation.

Maximal femur length must be preserved, because it will lessen the energy expenditure required for ambulation and improve the chances for the patient's successful rehabilitation. A circumferential skin incision is made 2 to 3 cm distal to the site of division of the femur (Fig. 15-7, *A* and *B*), ensuring that it is proximal to the patella and femoral condyles. Following division of the greater saphenous vein, the anterior and medial muscle groups are divided using electrocautery. The femoral artery and veins are suture ligated and the remaining musculature divided. The sciatic nerve is identified posteriorly and is dissected free; gentle traction is used, and the nerve is suture ligated and allowed to retract. Excessive traction on the sciatic nerve will result in a great deal of postoperative discomfort. The femur is then scored with electrocautery

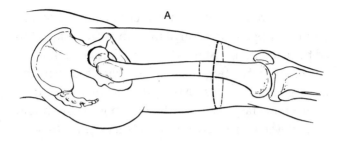

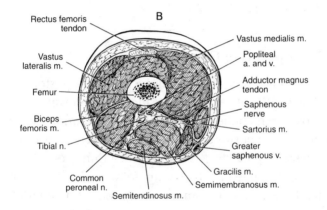

Rectus femoris tendon

Vastus lateralis m.

Femur

Biceps femoris m.

Tibial n.

Common peroneal n.

Semitendinosus m.

Vastus medialis m.

Popliteal a. and v.

Adductor magnus tendon

Saphenous nerve

Sartorius m.

Greater saphenous v.

Gracilis m.

Semimembranosus m.

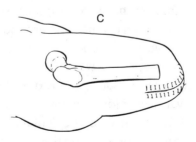

Fig. 15-7. A, Cross-sectional view of thigh at level of skin incision. **B,** Anatomic cross-sectional detail at level of skin incision. **C,** Skin closure of above-knee amputation.

2 to 3 cm proximal to the skin incision and the periosteum is stripped. Division of the femur can be facilitated by placing a moist towel over the proximal musculature and retracting these tissues with a pie-shaped tissue guard. The edges of the femur are then smoothed with a bone rasp. Hemostasis at the bone edge should be achieved with electrocautery rather than with bone wax. The wound is irrigated and closed as previously described (Fig. 15-7, *C*).

Postoperative Considerations

Major amputations may be managed postoperatively with soft or rigid dressings. Rigid dressings are most often applied to below-knee amputations as an immediate postoperative prosthesis (IPOP). Once the operative procedure is completed, a thin sheet of silk mesh is applied to the stump, followed by a layer of lamb's wool and a Spandex stump sock. Pads are then placed over bony prominences and a plaster or fiberglass cast is applied that incorporates a suspension strap with a belt which can be worn around the waist. An attachment plate is incorporated into the end portion of the stump cast into which a prosthesis can be fitted. Advantages include less postoperative stump swelling, prevention of joint flexion contractures and protection of the stump from incidental trauma. If an IPOP is used, there is the additional advantage of early ambulation. Disadvantages of IPOPs are that one is unable to inspect the wound during the 2 to 3 weeks that the rigid dressing remains in place, and there is some loss of joint mobility. A prosthetist must be available when the initial dressing is applied in the operating room. The most commonly used postoperative amputation dressing is the soft stump wrap. Gauze pads or *fluffs* are applied to the wound, followed by a gauze wrap and an elastic bandage. The amputation stump should be elevated to help reduce swelling. Critics of this technique cite the fact that edema may be poorly controlled, knee flexion contractures are not prevented, and stump maturity is necessary before the patient can ambulate, thereby prolonging the time required for rehabilitation. Nevertheless, the soft dressing is easy to apply, a rigid external knee splint will prevent most contractures, and a prosthetist need not be available for dressing changes. Early involvement of the physical therapist, preferably in the preoperative period, is crucial to achieving a good outcome with both techniques.

Overview of Rehabilitation

TOE OR RAY AMPUTATION. A prosthesis is not required. If the great toe has been amputated, a specially designed shoe constructed by an orthotist may be advantageous in improving balance.

TRANSMETATARSAL AMPUTATION. An orthotic shoe will assist in ambulation as well as in preventing trauma and subsequent breakdown of the transmetatarsal stump.

SYME'S AMPUTATION. Rehabilitation potential is very good; the patient requires a prosthetic device for out-of-the-home ambulation. There is approximately a 10% increase in energy expenditure necessary to ambulate, which most patients are able to tolerate.

BELOW-KNEE AMPUTATION. A 40% to 60% increase in energy expenditure is necessary for the patient to ambulate with a below-knee amputation. Nevertheless, the vast majority of patients who are ambulatory before amputation will achieve successful rehabilitation. Even with bilateral amputations, approximately 50% of patients will regain ambulatory ability.

ABOVE-KNEE AMPUTATION. Only one half of patients with an above-knee amputation are able to ambulate, principally because of the significant increase in energy expenditure necessary for ambulation, which may be more than 100% greater than normal. Rehabilitation potential with bilateral above-knee amputations is less than 5%. Wheelchair use alone requires a 9% increase in energy cost over normal ambulation.

Postoperative Complications

The reported incidence of ***phantom limb pain*** and ***disabling stump pain*** is 5% to 30%. These pain syndromes develop more commonly in patients following amputation for trauma and are difficult to treat. The principal means for avoiding significant, prolonged postoperative pain is aggressive rehabilitation, which can reduce the incidence to less than 5%. ***Hematoma*** formation can be avoided by meticulous intraoperative hemostasis. Occasionally closed suction drains may be indicated, but routine use of drains is not advocated. Perioperative antibiotic prophylaxis is appropriate to minimize postoperative infection, which has been reported in 12% to 28% of major amputations. Infection may necessitate revision of an amputation to a higher level. Mortality rates following major amputation have been reported to be as high as 10% for below-knee and 40% for above-knee amputations. The cause of such excessive mortality is often the underlying coronary artery disease present in these patients.

BIBLIOGRAPHY

Durham JR. Lower extremity amputation levels: Indications, methods of determining appropriate level, technique, prognosis. In Rutherford RB, ed. Vascular Surgery, 3rd ed. Philadelphia: WB Saunders, 1989, p 1687.

Epps CH, Jr. Amputation of the lower limb. In Evarts CM, ed. Surgery of the Musculoskeletal System. New York: Churchill Livingstone, 1990, pp 512-516.

Malone JM, Goldstone J. Lower extremity amputation. In Moore WS, ed. Vascular Surgery: A Comprehensive Review, 3rd ed. Philadelphia: WB Saunders, 1991, p 699.

Ouriel K, Fiore WM, Geary JE. Limb-threatening ischemia in the medically compromised patient: Amputation or revascularization? Surgery 104:667-672, 1988.

Piotrowski JJ, Bernhard VM. Noninvasive methods of determining amputation levels. In Ernst CB, Stanley JC, eds. Current Therapy in Vascular Surgery, 2nd ed. Philadelphia: BC Decker, 1991, p 690.

Samson RH, Gupta SK, Scher LA, Veith FJ. Level of amputation after failure of limb salvage procedures. Surg Gynecol Obstet 154:56-60, 1982.

Veith FJ, Gupta SK, Wengerter KR, Goldsmith J, Rivers SP, Bakal CW, Dietzek AM, Cynamon J, Sprayregen S, Gliedman ML. Changing arteriosclerotic disease patterns and management strategies in lower limb threatening ischemia. Ann Surg 4:402-414, 1990.

16

Hemodialysis Access

Ross T. Lyon • Ben U. Marsan

Access Planning and Timing of Placement

Although little interest is generated by hemodialysis access procedures, the importance of choosing the correct procedure cannot be overemphasized. Hemodialysis access is a lifesaving procedure, and, if done correctly, can permit the patient to have years of trouble-free therapy. When little attention is given to choosing an access site correctly or when operative technique is not meticulous, wasted access sites and the need for additional operative procedures are the result.

Acute renal failure frequently occurs without warning and often resolves without the need for extended hemodialysis access. Therefore temporary hemodialysis access with a percutaneously placed catheter is preferred as it can be used immediately and can be easily placed, changed, and removed as dictated by the clinical situation. Again, careful attention to detail is imperative if one is to avoid complications such as pneumothorax, sepsis, and impeded flow.

In patients with chronic progressive renal dysfunction, dialysis access planning should begin early, and efforts should be made to preserve the superficial veins of the upper extremities. Indwelling intravenous catheters and venipunctures, even for blood drawing, should be limited to veins on the dorsum of the hand. Long-term hemodialysis access should usually be established once the serum creatinine rises to 6 mg/dl or the creatinine clearance falls to 10 ml/min. This will usually allow enough time for the access site to "mature" before use. If access procedures are postponed until dialysis is needed, both acute and chronic access procedures will be necessary to allow immediate dialysis as well as to provide a long-term access site that can mature before use.

Terminology

A *dialysis catheter* is a large-bore dual-lumen central venous catheter that is usually inserted percutaneously. One port serves as the outflow (to the dialysis machine) and the other port as the inflow (to the patient from the machine).

An *arteriovenous fistula* consists of an anastomosis of an autologous artery to an adjacent superficial vein. This produces a high-flow circuit, resulting in dilation of a superficial vein, which can be percutaneously cannulated for hemodialysis access. This is to be distinguished from an *arteriovenous graft*, which is the interposition of a vascular conduit (such as those made from polytetrafluoroethylene [PTFE] or bovine carotid artery) between an artery (inflow) and a vein (outflow). The graft itself is punctured to establish dialysis access. Both of these arteriovenous communications differ from an *arteriovenous shunt* which involves an *externalized* communication between the arterial and venous circulation. This generally is composed of Silastic tubing with one end connected to an artery and the other to a vein. Continuity of flow is established by a connector that is removed to allow each limb to be temporarily connected to the dialysis machine. This modality is rarely used since the development of temporary dialysis catheters that can be rapidly inserted percutaneously.

Access Axioms

Effective hemodialysis requires high flow rates into and out of the dialyzer (300 to 400 ml/min). Therefore arterialized veins, resilient prosthetic grafts, or large central veins are required for hemodialysis access. All access sites must be located superficially to allow for simple percutaneous puncture. To avoid injury, these sites should *not* be near vital structures such as major nerves or arteries. Since hemodialysis access sites have a finite life-span, the use of the more distal extremity is initially preferred to preserve the latter for subsequent use. *Upper* extremity placement is certainly recommended rather than the use of the lower extremity, because it presents an easier access site and has lower rates of infection. Autologous fistulas are preferred to implanted grafts because of their superior patency rate and lower complication rate.

Acute Dialysis Access Options

DIRECT SINGLE-LUMEN PERCUTANEOUS PUNC-TURES. Simultaneous femoral artery and vein punctures may be used in patients with no existing dialysis access. However, this technique poses the significant risk of developing a groin hematoma or serious vessel injury (thrombosis, pseudoaneurysm, or arteriovenous [AV] fistula formation).

NONCUFFED DUAL-LUMEN DIALYSIS CATHETERS. Percutaneous placement of a dual-lumen dialysis catheter (Fig. 16-1, *A*) (Shiley, Quinton, or VasCath catheters) is a simple bedside procedure for temporary hemodialysis access. This technique, using the sterile Seldinger method, allows access in an emergency setting without the need for transporting the patient to the operating room. These catheters may be used for up to 2 months if no signs of infection or central vein thrombosis develop. Attention to detail is important in these patients to avoid the complications of pneumothorax, inadvertent arterial cannulation, or infection.

CUFFED DIALYSIS CATHETERS. Placement of a *cuffed dialysis catheter* (Fig. 16-1, *B*) (PermCath or VasCath catheter) generally requires a venous cutdown technique, although it may be achieved percutaneously with only a small incision. These catheters may be used immediately, and their softer material is better

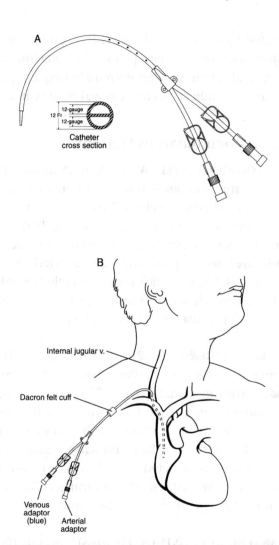

A

12-gauge
12 Fr
12-gauge
Catheter
cross section

B

Internal jugular v.

Dacron felt cuff

Venous
adaptor
(blue)

Arterial
adaptor

Fig. 16-1. A, Noncuffed dual-lumen dialysis catheter. **B,** Cuffed dialysis catheter.

tolerated by patients and allows the catheter to remain in place for prolonged periods. Catheter infection and central venous thrombosis remain frequent problems and are indications for removal of the catheter.

Chronic Hemodialysis Options

AUTOLOGOUS ARTERIOVENOUS DIALYSIS FISTULAS. A direct arteriovenous fistula of an upper extremity artery to a superficial vein will usually result in the most trouble-free chronic dialysis access. Three-year patency rates for autologous arteriovenous dialysis fistulas are 70% compared with 55% for arteriovenous access grafts. The complication rates (including infection and pseudoaneurysm formation) are considerably lower for fistulas than for AV grafts.

WRIST FISTULA (Fig. 16-2). If the superficial veins are adequate and the arterial inflow to the hand is normal, a radial artery to cephalic vein AV fistula (AVF) should be constructed in the nondominant arm as the initial access procedure in a patient with end-stage renal disease. This fistula is called a *Brescia-Cimino fistula* and is usually constructed as a side-to-side anastomosis with the vein distal to the anastomosis ligated to avoid venous hypertension of the hand.

ANTECUBITAL FISTULA (Fig. 16-3). The superficial veins are often inadequate for use in a wrist fistula— usually because of multiple previous venipunctures.

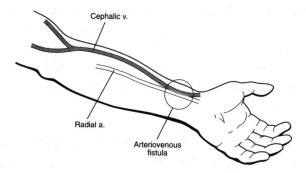

Fig. 16-2. Wrist fistula (left arm).

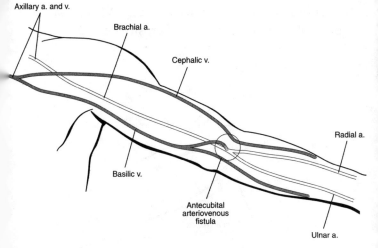

Fig. 16-3. Antecubital fistula.

In these cases, the antecubital or cephalic vein at the level of the antecubital fossa may remain adequate for a primary AVF. There must be enough length of cephalic vein proximal to the fistula to allow for multiple cannulation sites. Care must be taken to ligate adjacent tributaries that could permit venous outflow via the deep veins.

TRANSPOSED VEIN ARTERIOVENOUS FISTULAS (Fig. 16-4). If the superficial veins are atrophic or obliterated, the brachial or basilic vein of the upper arm can be mobilized, tunneled subcutaneously, and anastomosed to the brachial artery to allow an autologous upper extremity dialysis access to develop. This option is inferior to a standard nontransposed AVF but may be preferable, in some cases, to a prosthetic graft.

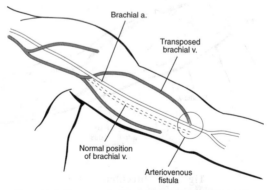

Fig. 16-4. Transposed vein arteriovenous fistula.

DIALYSIS ACCESS GRAFTS. When the superficial veins of the arms are not satisfactory to allow a functional autologous AV dialysis fistula to develop, a prosthetic AV graft is used to establish long-term hemodialysis access. These prosthetic access grafts are inferior to autologous fistulas because of their higher rates of thrombosis, infection and pseudoaneurysm formation. Similar principles for graft placement apply in that the initial access grafts should be placed *distally* in the arm to preserve the more proximal veins for future access procedures. The choice of graft material varies among surgeons but may include PTFE, tanned bovine carotid artery, or cryopreserved veins.

FOREARM ARTERIOVENOUS GRAFTS. A *straight fore-arm graft* (Fig. 16-5) represents the most straightforward type of dialysis access graft. This graft extends from the radial artery (at the level of the wrist) to a vein in the antecubital fossa (the basilic, cephalic, or ante-brachial vein). The difficulties encountered with the straight graft are its very limited area for puncture sites and the reported decrease in patency rates when compared with the loop configuration. All forearm grafts performed in patients with diabetes may be complicated by a heavily calcified radial artery, which may not provide for high enough flow to maintain graft patency.

A *forearm loop graft* (Fig. 16-6) is constructed from the distal brachial artery to a vein in the antecubital fossa. However, the course of the graft begins at the

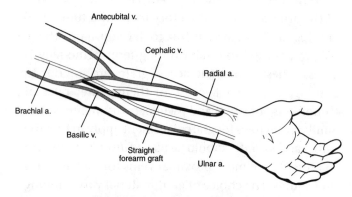

Fig. 16-5. Straight forearm graft.

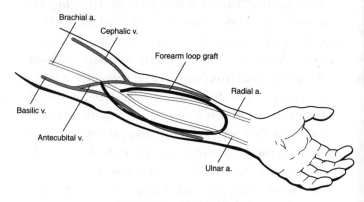

Fig. 16-6. Forearm loop graft.

arterial anastomosis, tracks distally in a carefully created subcutaneous tunnel, and returns to the venous anastomosis after a gentle "U-turn" is created in the distal forearm. This configuration provides for superior inflow (the flow into the graft is in the *same* direction as the native arterial flow) and greater usable length for punctures. This graft is technically more demanding and requires care to avoid angulation or kinking.

UPPER ARM GRAFTS. These grafts are placed when the vessels of the forearm have been utilized for previous access grafts or are unusable. A *curved upper arm graft* (Fig. 16-7) is one that originates from the brachial artery near the antecubital fossa, is tunneled subcutaneously over the dorsal and lateral aspects of the upper arm, and is anastomosed to the cephalic, basilic, or axillary vein in the proximal portion of the upper extremity. It is possible to place the graft in a "reversed" orientation extending from the axillary artery in the upper arm to the brachial vein at the level of the antecubital fossa. The arterial inflow and venous outflow are usually sufficient for this type of graft, except in the presence of a recent subclavian vein thrombosis.

A *looped upper arm graft* (Fig. 16-8) uses the distal portion of the axillary artery and vein. Much like a forearm loop, the looped upper arm graft is placed in a subcutaneous tunnel with the curve extending just proximal to the antecubital fossa.

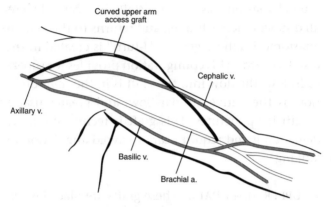

Fig. 16-7. Curved upper arm graft.

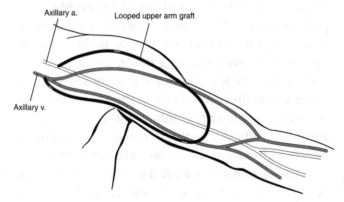

Fig. 16-8. Looped upper arm graft.

CHRONIC DIALYSIS CATHETERS. A cuffed dialysis catheter (Fig. 16-1, *B*) is a dual-lumen catheter that may be placed either percutaneously into a central vein (internal jugular or subclavian) or by a cutdown technique into the upper cephalic or jugular vein. Recurrent catheter thrombosis remains a common problem but may be treated by injecting 5000 to 10,000 U of urokinase into each catheter lumen. Low or intermittent flow, central vein thrombosis, and catheter infection are other complications associated with this technique of hemodialysis access.

Preoperative Assessment and Care

ASSESSMENT OF SUPERFICIAL VEINS IN CHOOSING AN OPERATIVE PROCEDURE. Venous outflow is frequently the limiting factor associated with establishing and maintaining hemodialysis access. Therefore careful examination of the superficial arm veins is the single most important part of the evaluation before deciding on a dialysis access procedure. Distended or tortuous superficial veins or the presence of a swollen arm suggest a proximal venous obstruction. A venogram, or careful duplex evaluation, should be performed before use of that arm for hemodialysis access, since a proximal venous (outflow) obstruction would doom the graft to early failure.

The superficial veins of the arm are most easily examined after placing a tourniquet around the upper arm. If the cephalic vein is palpated at the wrist and is ballottable up to the level of the antecubital fossa, a primary AV wrist fistula between the cephalic vein and the radial artery should be the initial access procedure (Brescia-Cimino fistula). When the forearm veins are obliterated or atrophic but the antecubital and cephalic veins are ballottable, an antecubital AVF (brachial artery to antecubital or cephalic vein) is desirable. If the basilic vein is prominent and patent down to the level of the wrist, then an ulnar artery to basilic vein AVF should be considered. The absence of any visible superficial upper extremity veins mandates the consideration of other less durable access procedures.

PROTECTION OF SUPERFICIAL UPPER EXTREMITY VEINS. Because of the importance of the superficial upper extremity veins in establishing and maintaining chronic hemodialysis access, these veins should be "protected" in patients with impending or established renal failure. Venipuncture of these veins (for blood drawing or intravenous line placement) should be strictly prohibited by written orders for hospitalized patients. Venous access for blood drawing or fluid administration should be limited to the veins in the dorsum of the hands except in emergency situations.

ASSESSMENT OF ARTERIAL INFLOW. Placement of an AV graft or fistula in an extremity with compromised arterial inflow can result in premature occlusion, failure of a fistula to mature, or ischemia of the extremity as a result of an arterial steal syndrome. Arterial inflow can usually be assessed by palpating peripheral pulses or comparing the extremity blood pressure with that in the contralateral arm. Diminished pulses or a 10 mm Hg difference in systolic blood pressure suggests arterial compromise and is a contraindication to graft or fistula placement.

Operative Considerations

AV fistula operations can usually be performed using only local anesthesia, whereas prosthetic graft placement may require a regional block. Preoperative antibiotics (usually vancomycin) are administered before placement of a prosthetic graft. Gentle handling of the tissues is important to avoid wound breakdown and possible secondary graft infection. Grafts should be placed superficially in the subcutaneous tissue to allow for percutaneous cannulation. Care must be taken to avoid vessel or graft angulation, kinking, or twists, which are likely to cause thrombosis. Attention to hemostasis and avoidance of wound and perigraft hematomas are important to preventing wound breakdown, infection, and graft occlusion.

Postoperative Evaluation and Care

POSTOPERATIVE CHECK. Graft or fistula patency should be confirmed by the presence of a palpable thrill at the venous anastomosis. Distal perfusion should be confirmed by the presence of distal pulses, demonstrating adequate capillary refill and assessing the skin temperature of both the involved and the contralateral extremities. Symptoms of ischemic rest pain or pain on exercise are infrequently reported by patients. Neurologic function must also be assessed to exclude severe distal ischemia resulting from an arterial occlusion or steal syndrome.

The arm should be elevated above the level of the heart in the early postoperative period to minimize the edema that is common with forearm grafts. Circumferential dressings should be avoided because of a possible tourniquet effect. Significant local wound hematomas should be identified early and evacuated in the operating room. Range of motion exercises of the fingers and hand are begun on the first postoperative day so as to avoid stiffness.

FISTULA AND GRAFT MATURATION. Hemodialysis fistulas and grafts should be allowed to mature before they are used. A 2-week period will generally suffice to allow for the fibrous adherence of the graft to the surrounding tissues. This fibrous encapsulation of the graft assists in decreasing the incidence of a perigraft hematoma (with subsequent infection) or graft thrombosis precipitated by early graft puncture. AVFs require a 2- to 3-month period to allow for dilatation and thickening of the arterialized veins. This enables a more effective percutaneous cannulation and minimizes the chance of occlusion of the cannulated vein. The following often lead to maturation failure of the AVF:

- Proximal or distal arterial stenosis
- Inadequate outflow veins or stenosis in the veins cephalad to the venous anastomosis
- Presence of a perforating vein that diverts fistula flow into the deep veins

CARE OF DIALYSIS ACCESS GRAFTS. Puncture sites in dialysis grafts should be distributed along the length of the graft or arterialized vein. This requires that the cannulation sites be rotated by the hemodialysis nurse to minimize the likelihood of pseudoaneurysm formation or focal stenosis and subsequent graft failure. Strict adherence to sterile technique is necessary to minimize the possibilities of infectious complications. Careful cannulation technique must be employed to avoid perforation of the posterior wall of the graft, which can cause perigraft hematomas. Attention to the systemic blood pressure during the hemodialysis run is imperative to avoid prolonged periods of hypotension that may render the graft susceptible to occlusion. Appropriate pressure must be applied following removal of the access needles to avoid both pseudoaneurysm formation (too little pressure or too short a duration) and graft thrombosis (excessive pressure).

Common Dialysis Access Problems

CATHETER-INDUCED CENTRAL VEIN THROMBOSIS. Indwelling temporary and long-term central venous dialysis catheters act as a nidus for thrombus formation, with symptomatic central venous thrombosis occurring in 7% to 20% of these patients. Thrombosis can be limited to the catheter itself or it may result in a fibrin sheath forming around the catheter. Thrombosis of the subclavian or internal jugular veins or of the superior vena cava is a much more serious complication. In the absence of central vein thrombosis, a thrombosed dialysis access catheter can occasionally be salvaged by injecting 5000 to 10,000 U of urokinase into each catheter port to reestablish catheter patency. New onset of extremity edema or poor catheter flow rates suggest central venous thrombosis. Treatment of symptomatic central venous thrombosis consists of catheter removal, temporary systemic anticoagulation therapy, and arm elevation until the edema has resolved. Future dialysis access procedures should avoid the use of the affected arm because of the likelihood of subsequent arm edema.

POORLY FUNCTIONING FISTULA OR GRAFT. Maximal dialysis flow rates of less than 300 ml/min, recirculation rates higher than 15%, or venous pressures greater than 150 mm Hg indicate access malfunction. A patent but poorly functioning fistula or graft usually results from an obstructing lesion of the venous outflow tract but can also be caused by a stenosis of the arterial inflow or of the graft itself. Prominent pulsations in the graft or fistula suggest proximal venous obstruction, whereas decreased pulsations or a thrill suggest an inflow stenosis. Angiography of the associated vessels and graft (a *fistulogram*) should be obtained to define and accurately localize the problem. Most lesions affecting the function of the graft or fistula should be corrected by operative repair; however, selected focal lesions may respond to balloon angioplasty.

ACUTE OCCLUSION OF DIALYSIS FISTULA OR GRAFT. Perioperative occlusion of an AVF is unusual but may result from an unrecognized outflow stenosis or a technical imperfection in the construction of the anastomosis. Differentiating between these two possible causes is difficult in the clinical setting and will require prompt reexploration, thrombectomy, and intraoperative venography to elucidate the cause. This aggressive approach, with revision of either the anastomosis or outflow site, is necessary to salvage the fistula for later use.

Graft occlusion in the immediate postoperative period is usually caused by a technical problem such as a graft kink, thrombus deposition at the time of surgery, or use of an inadequate outflow vein. Grafts occluding in the immediate postoperative period should be reexplored and revised based on intraoperative findings. An intraoperative arteriogram and venogram should be obtained following thrombectomy if the problem is not obvious. Other causes of failure of newly placed grafts include graft infection, systemic hypotension, and hypercoagulability.

LATE GRAFT OR FISTULA OCCLUSION. Dialysis fistulas often become dysfunctional ("failing graft") before occluding. Much like grafts in the peripheral arterial circulation, intervention on a failing dialysis graft can extend its patency over that of a graft that requires thrombectomy because of occlusion. When a recent thrombosis of the graft occurs, urokinase thrombolysis by way of percutaneously placed catheters will often reestablish patency and uncover the lesion responsible for the occlusion. Correction of the underlying lesion, either by operative or interventional techniques, is necessary to maintain patency. Chronic occlusions render an AVF unsalvageable.

Late graft occlusions are often the result of perianastomotic neointimal hyperplasia involving the venous outflow of the graft. This occurs most commonly from 6 months to 2 years following graft placement. Occlusions occurring later than 2 years after graft placement are usually the result of intragraft lesions from fibrous ingrowth into closely spaced puncture sites. Both of these lesions are best repaired by short interposition grafts bypassing the obstructed segment.

ARTERIAL STEAL SYNDROME. The low-resistance venous outflow of AVFs and grafts may result in a steal phenomenon in which distal perfusion of the extremity is compromised by the shunting of arterial flow into the low-resistance fistula or graft. This problem worsens over time as the outflow tract matures and develops compensatory dilatation. A steal syndrome is especially likely if there is an arterial stenosis proximal to the fistula or graft. Absent distal pulses and decreased distal perfusion that normalize with temporary manual compression of the fistula or graft are diagnostic of a steal phenomenon. Symptoms of the steal syndrome may include a cold hand and occasional paresthesias in mild cases, and ischemic rest pain in severe cases. If untreated, the arterial steal may lead to finger necrosis or sustained neurologic dysfunction. Treatment consists of banding or ligating the fistula or the proximal outflow tract of the graft.

HIGH-FLOW ARTERIOVENOUS FISTULAS. Autologous AV dialysis fistulas occasionally allow excessive flow rates that may have adverse systemic consequences such as tachycardia, congestive heart failure, and even hypertrophic cardiomyopathy. Prosthetic grafts rarely cause these problems because of the fixed flow resistance of the graft itself. Correction of high-flow states requires banding or obliteration of the fistula or graft.

INFECTION. Autologous dialysis fistulas rarely become primarily infected. Secondary infection of an AVF is more common and is usually the result of contiguous spread of an infection of a hematoma surrounding the fistula. Contrariwise, dialysis catheter and graft infections are relatively common. These access infections are often caused by a break in sterile techniques, which thereby allows the introduction of *Staphylococcus aureus* or *S. epidermidis* organisms from skin. The frequency of catheter infection is inversely related to the quality of the local care of the catheter. Catheter exit sites should be cleaned daily, painted with an antiseptic solution, and covered with a dry gauze dressing. Transparent plastic occlusive dressings should be avoided, because they promote underlying bacterial growth. Catheter infections can occasionally be resolved with intravenous administration of antibiotics, but they frequently recur and are best treated by removal of the catheter.

Infection involving dialysis access grafts occasionally occurs at the time of surgery but usually results from contamination during cannulation for dialysis, especially if multiple punctures and perigraft hematomas occur. Early postoperative cellulitis can occasionally be treated with intravenous antibiotics, but persistent cellulitis is usually the result of graft infection. Overtly infected dialysis grafts, when the entire graft is involved, should be entirely excised and the skin left open temporarily until the infection has resolved. Infection may present as a thrombosed graft that on exploration is not well incorporated by ingrowth of the surrounding tissues. When this situation is encountered, the graft should be presumed to be infected and should therefore be removed. Occasionally an abscess or cellulitis adjacent to but involving only a portion of the graft or the anastomotic sites can be treated without graft excision if the localized infection is adequately drained and intravenous antibiotics are administered.

ANEURYSMS AND PSEUDOANEURYSMS. Aneurysmal changes of autologous AVFs and pseudoaneurysms in dialysis grafts are fairly common. The dilatation seen with autologous fistulas is initially a compensatory change in vessel diameter because of high flow velocities and turbulence. This aneurysmal change involves all layers of the vessel wall and is usually self limiting or only slowly progressive. Surgical obliteration of these lesions is usually not necessary unless the overlying skin has thinned enough that external rupture is possible. The focal dilatations seen with dialysis grafts, however, are actually pseudoaneurysms resulting from multiple closely spaced puncture sites. The wall of these lesions consists only of organized thrombus and subcutaneous tissues. Graft pseudoaneurysms are progressive lesions that can continue to expand until erosion and rupture through the skin occurs resulting in massive hemorrhage and possible exsanguination. Therefore graft pseudoaneurysms should be repaired early by exclusion with a short segment graft interposition.

BIBLIOGRAPHY

Bell DD, Rosenthal JJ. Arteriovenous graft life in chronic hemodialysis: A need for prolongation. Arch Surg 123:1169-1172, 1988.

Bhat DJ, Tellis VA, Kohlberg WI, Driscoll B, Veith FJ. Management of sepsis involving expanded polytetrafluoroethylene grafts for hemodialysis access. Surgery 87:445-450, 1980.

Dunea G, Domenico L, Gunnerson P, Winston-Willis F. A survey of permanent double lumen catheters in hemodialysis patients. ASAIO Trans 37:M276-M277, 1991.

Levy SS, Sherman RA, Nosher SL. Value of clinical screening for detection of asymptomatic hemodialysis vascular access stenoses. Angiology 43:421-424, 1992.

Mattson WJ. Recognition and treatment of vascular steal secondary to hemodialysis prostheses. Am J Surg 154:198-201, 1987.

Palder SB, Kirkman RL, Whittemore AD, Hakim RM, Lazarus JM, Tilney NL. Vascular access for hemodialysis patency rates and results of revision. Ann Surg 202:235-239, 1985.

Raju S. PTFE Grafts for hemodialysis access. Techniques for insertion and management of complications. Ann Surg 206(5):666-673, 1987.

Rivers SP, Scher LA, Sheehan E, Lynn R, Veith FJ. Basilic vein transposition: An underused autologous alternative to prosthetic dialysis angioaccess. J Vasc Surg 18:391-397, 1993.

Tordoir JH, Herman JM, Kwan TS, Diderich PM. Long-term follow-up of the polytetrafluoroethylene (PTFE) prosthesis as an arteriovenous fistula for hemodialysis. Europ J Vasc Surg. 2:3-7, 1988.

Wilson ES. Vascular Access Surgery. Chicago: Year Book, 1988.

Zibari GB, Rohr MS, Landreneau MD, Bridges RM, DeVault GA, Petty FH, Costley KJ, Brown ST, McDonald JC. Complications from permanent hemodialysis vascular access. Surgery 104:681-686, 1988.

Appendix

Preoperative Checklist

A. *Summary*
   1. Concisely document a description of patient's pertinent history with specific attention to indications for operation
   2. Indicate the alternatives to surgery and their disadvantages
   3. Enter notation that the alternatives to surgery and all of the risks of the surgical procedure have been discussed with the patient (and family); be sure to indicate that the patient has voiced a clear understanding of the planned procedure and its risks and benefits

B. *Data Consolidation*
   This part of the record should include all of the pertinent data that will be needed by the surgeon and anesthesiologist performing the operation
   1. Planned procedure (*including* the side of the body!)
   2. Preoperative diagnosis and comorbid medical illness
   3. Current relevant medications (insulin, cardiac medications, antihypertensives, and steroids)
   4. Laboratory values
      a. Chemistry (including creatinine)
      b. Complete blood count (with platelet count)

    c. Coagulation profile
      (1) Prothrombin time
      (2) Partial thromboplastin time
      (3) Bleeding time (if indicated)
    d. Urinalysis

5. Cardiac evaluation
    a. Name of cardiologist following patient
    b. Electrocardiogram
    c. Results of echocardiogram (if indicated)
    d. Results of cardiac workup (if this was performed)
      (1) Dipyridamole-thallium stress test
      (2) Cardiac catheterization
    e. Dates of prior coronary artery bypass surgery
    f. Swan-Ganz catheterization parameters (if indicated)
      (1) Initial values (pulmonary artery pressures, pulmonary capillary wedge pressure, central venous pressure, cardiac index, systemic vascular resistance)
      (2) Creation of Starling curve, noting optimal filling pressures

6. Pulmonary evaluation
    a. Name of pulmonologist following patient
    b. Results of most recent chest x-ray films
    c. Arterial blood gases (if indicated—COPD, aortic procedure, etc.)
    d. Results of pulmonary function testing (if indicated)

7. Endocrine evaluation
   a. Name of endocrinologist following patient
   b. Glucose levels on day of surgery
      (1) Ensure that insulin dose has been adjusted correctly
      (2) Glucose monitoring on day of surgery (especially for late cases)
8. Neurologic evaluation (carotid endarterectomies)
   a. Name of neurologist following patient
   b. Results of cerebral angiogram
   c. Results of most recent head CT scan or MRI
   d. Document any neurologic deficits
9. Medical clearance for major procedures
   a. Check with physician following patient
   b. List name of attending medical physician
10. Blood bank
    a. Ensure that specimen is in blood bank
    b. Verify availability of necessary blood products
11. Results of noninvasive laboratory evaluations
    a. Pulse volume recordings (revascularization and aortic procedures)
    b. Carotid duplex (carotid endarterectomy [CEA])
12. Informed consent
    a. Ensure that operative side indicated on consent is the side with the pathologic condition!
    b. Check dates and witnessed signatures

        c. For amputations, obtain consent for more extensive procedure than planned ("one level higher")

C. *Miscellaneous Considerations*

    1. Preoperative anesthesia consultation

        a. Patients at especially high risk

        b. Unusual surgical or anesthetic requirements

           (1) Previous difficult intubation

           (2) Family history of malignant hyperthermia

           (3) Unusual positioning of patient

    2. Special considerations for aortic procedures (aneurysmal and occlusive disease)

        a. Avoid administration of antiplatelet agents for 10 days before surgery

        b. Arrange for autologous blood transfusion, if possible

        c. Arrange for "cell saver" equipment

        d. Preoperative bowel preparation

           (1) Clear liquid diet for 24 hours preoperatively

           (2) Mechanical preparation on day before surgery

           (3) Antibiotic preparation (per surgeon's preference)

               (a) Enteral antibiotics (kanamycin and erythromycin base)

               (b) Parenteral antibiotics (cephalosporin) on day of operation

3. Special considerations for carotid endarterectomy procedures
   a. Begin antiplatelet therapy on night before surgery
   b. Thoroughly document an accurate neurologic examination

Postoperative Checklist

A. *Postoperative Orders*
   1. Documentation of procedure performed
   2. Bed rest for 24 hours (at least)
   3. Neurovascular checks hourly for the initial 24 hours
   4. Intravenous fluids
      a. Careful consideration of fluid and rate
         (1) Diabetic patients
         (2) Poor cardiac reserve
         (3) Account for fluid administered in OR and blood loss
      b. Urine output may serve as guide
   5. Medications
      a. Review preoperative medications *carefully*
      b. Consider insulin requirements
      c. Stress doses of steroids if indicated
      d. Use of anticoagulants or antiplatelet agents
   6. Diet
      a. Begin slowly and advance as tolerated
      b. Aortic procedures generally require nasogastric drainage

          (1) Consider antacids or histamine blockers
          (2) Monitor gastric pH level
     7. Laboratory tests
       a. Recovery room
          (1) Complete blood count
          (2) SMA-6 and creatinine
          (3) Cardiac enzymes
          (4) Electrocardiogram
          (5) Chest x-ray films
       b. Early postoperative period
          (1) Follow hematocrit
          (2) Electrolytes daily
          (3) Cardiac enzymes (three sets postoperatively, if results are all negative)
          (4) Electrocardiogram daily
          (5) Medication levels (digoxin, theophylline, procainamide, etc.)
     8. Document pulse examination at end of operation
     9. No constrictive stockings or antiembolism devices on lower extremities following arterial bypass surgery
B. *Initial Postoperative Visit*
     1. Ideally, 6 hours after procedure
     2. Recheck orders for completeness and accuracy (especially medications)
     3. Evaluate hemodynamic status
       a. Urine output
       b. Swan-Ganz catheter profile
     4. Evaluate respiratory status

a. Postoperative chest x-ray films
b. If patient is intubated, evaluate endotracheal tube position
c. Respiratory efforts
d. Effects of sedation (narcotics)
e. Arterial blood gases, if indicated

5. Neurologic evaluation
   a. Detailed examination to include cranial nerves following CEA
   b. Assess mental status
      (1) If altered, consider cardiopulmonary etiology *first*
      (2) Narcotic administration parenterally or via epidural catheter

6. Review postoperative laboratory tests
7. Document pulse examination (and compare with preoperative and intraoperative)
8. Assess dressings for excess drainage
9. Infected and contaminated wounds should be redressed on first postoperative day

Angiography Protocol

A. *Preangiography Checklist*
   1. Summary
      a. Concise description of pertinent history, with specific attention to angiography
      b. Notation that the risks and benefits of angiography have been discussed and *are understood* by patient and family

2. Laboratory data
   a. SMA-6 and creatinine
   b. Complete blood count with platelet count
   c. Coagulation profile
      (1) Prothrombin time
      (2) Partial thromboplastin time
      (3) Bleeding time (if indicated)
   d. Electrocardiogram
   e. Chest x-ray films
3. Allergy to contrast material, iodine, or shellfish
   a. Note previous reaction (exact manifestations)
   b. Consider use of steroids, antihistamine, or general anesthesia
4. Specimen to blood bank for blood typing
5. Intravenous hydration begun evening before angiogram (if inpatient)
6. Nothing to eat or drink for 8 hours before examination
   a. Adjust insulin dosing
   b. Hold oral hypoglycemic medications
   c. Intravenous glucose administration
7. Renal insufficiency
   a. Consider mannitol and/or lasix
   b. Careful hydration
8. Hypertension
   a. Ensure that patient receives antihypertensive medications before procedure

b. Hypertensive episodes can increase bleeding complications

9. Preparation of groin as indicated

10. Obtain informed consent per institutional protocol

B. *Postangiography Checklist*

1. Initial visit should be shortly after procedure, with subsequent visit 6 hours later

2. Bed rest immediately following procedure (length varies by institution)

3. Examine puncture site for mass (hematoma versus pseudoaneurysm)

4. Examine pulse carefully

5. Administer intravenous hydration as tolerated
   a. Maintain adequate urine output
   b. Assess for impending congestive heart failure

6. Follow electrolytes and renal function after procedure

7. Clinical assessment of retroperitoneum for occult hemorrhage
   a. Serial hematocrit tests if bleeding is suspected
   b. Follow white blood cell count
   c. Emergent CT scan

8. Intra-arterial urokinase infusion
   a. Patient must be in monitored setting
   b. Careful monitoring of laboratory values

Arterial and Venous Anatomy

KEY: a., artery; aa., arteries; m., muscle; n., nerve; v., vein; ant., anterior; ext., external; inf., inferior; int., internal; lat., lateral; med., medial; post., posterior; sup., superior.

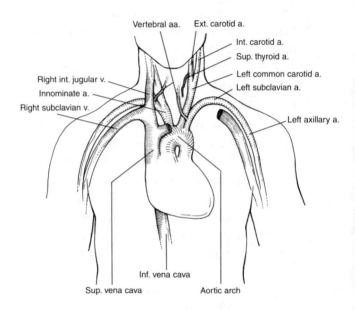

Fig. A-1. The great vessels and aortic arch.

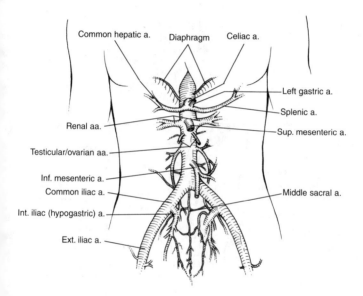

Fig. A-2. The abdominal aorta and its branches.

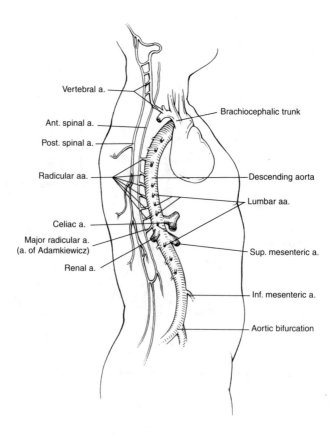

Fig. A-3. Descending aorta and its branches.

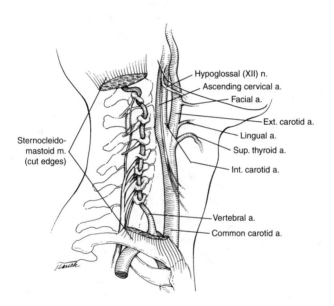

Fig. A-4. Cerebral blood supply.

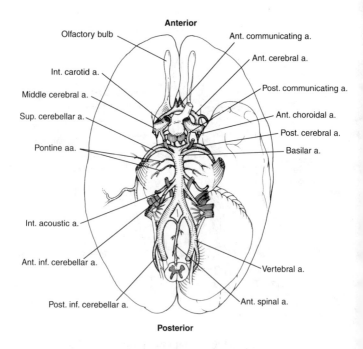

Fig. A-5. Intracerebral circulation (circle of Willis).

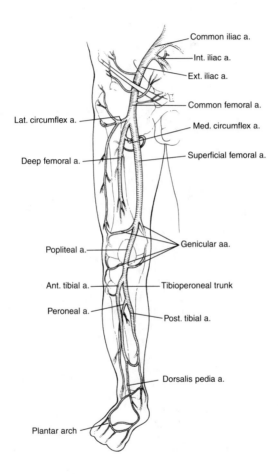

Fig. A-6. Arterial supply to the lower extremity.

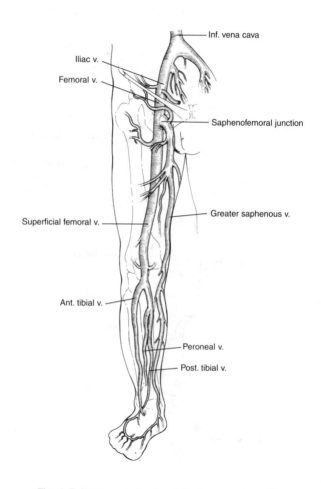

Fig. A-7. Venous drainage of the lower extremity.

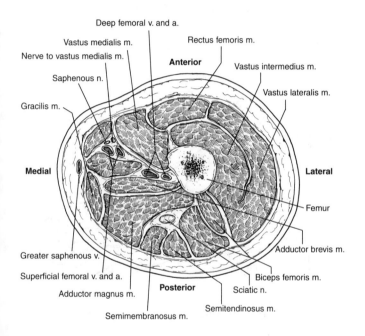

Fig. A-8. Cross section through the mid-femur.

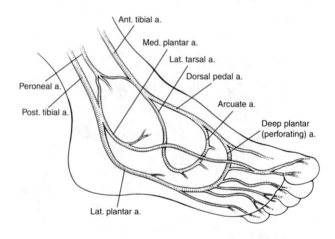

Fig. A-9. Arterial supply to the foot.

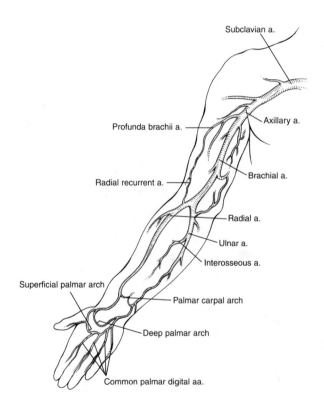

Fig. A-10. Arterial supply to the upper extremity.

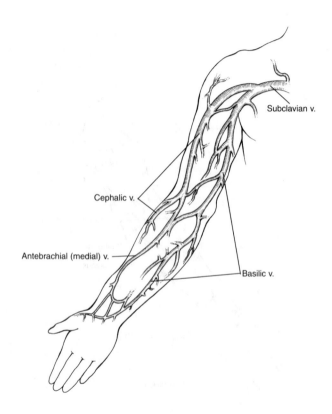

Subclavian v.

Cephalic v.

Antebrachial (medial) v.

Basilic v.

Fig. A-11. Venous drainage of the upper extremity.

Index